Psychotherapy for Personality Disorders

Review of Psychiatry Series
John M. Oldham, M.D., and
Michelle B. Riba, M.D.
Series Editors

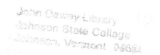
Psychotherapy for Personality Disorders

EDITED BY

John G. Gunderson, M.D.

Glen O. Gabbard, M.D.

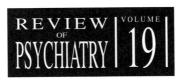

REVIEW OF PSYCHIATRY | VOLUME 19

No. 3

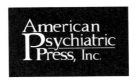

American Psychiatric Press, Inc.

Washington, DC
London, England

JE 21 '03

Note: The authors have worked to ensure that all information in this book concerning drug dosages, schedules, and routes of administration is accurate as of the time of publication and consistent with standards set by the U.S. Food and Drug Administration and the general medical community. As medical research and practice advance, however, therapeutic standards may change. For this reason and because human and mechanical errors sometimes occur, we recommend that readers follow the advice of a physician who is directly involved in their care or the care of a member of their family.

Books published by the American Psychiatric Press, Inc., represent the views and opinions of the individual authors and do not necessarily represent the policies and opinions of the Press or the American Psychiatric Association.

Copyright © 2000 American Psychiatric Press, Inc.

03   02   01   00   4   3   2   1

ALL RIGHTS RESERVED
Manufactured in the United States of America on acid-free paper

American Psychiatric Press, Inc.
1400 K Street, NW
Washington, DC 20005
www.appi.org

The correct citation for this book is

>   Gunderson JG, Gabbard GO (eds.): *Psychotherapy for Personality Disorders* (Review of Psychiatry Series, Vol. 19, No. 3; Oldham JO and Riba MB, series eds.). Washington, DC, American Psychiatric Press, 2000

Library of Congress Cataloging-in-Publication Data
Psychotherapy for personality disorders / edited by John G. Gunderson, Glen O. Gabbard.
>   p. ; cm. — (Review of psychiatry ; v. 19, no. 3)
>   Includes bibliographical references and index.
>   ISBN 0-88048-273-7 (alk. paper)
>   1. Personality disorders—Treatment. 2. Psychotherapy. I. Gunderson, John G., 1942–   . II. Gabbard, Glen O. III. Review of psychiatry series ; v. 19, 3
>   [DNLM: 1. Personality Disorders—therapy. 2. Psychotherapy—methods. WM 190 P9759 2000]
>   RC554.P78 2000
>   616.85´8—dc21

00-024853

British Library Cataloguing in Publication Data
A CIP record is available from the British Library.

Review of Psychiatry Series ISSN 1041-5882

Cover: Digital imagery © copyright 1999 PhotoDisc, Inc.

Contents

Contributors

Michael Bond, M.D.
Associate Professor of Psychiatry, McGill University; Psychiatrist-in-Chief, Institute of Community and Family Psychiatry, Sir Mortimer B. Davis–Jewish General Hospital, Montréal, Québec, Canada

Kate Davidson, Ph.D.
Research Tutor and Consultant Clinical Psychologist, Department of Psychological Medicine, University of Glasgow, Gartnavel Royal Hospital, Glasgow, Scotland

Glen O. Gabbard, M.D.
Callaway Distinguished Professor of Psychoanalysis and Education, Karl Menninger School of Psychiatry and Mental Health Sciences at The Menninger Clinic; Director and Training and Supervising Analyst, Topeka Institute for Psychoanalysis; Clinical Professor of Psychiatry, University of Kansas School of Medicine—Wichita

John G. Gunderson, M.D.
Director of Psychotherapy and Psychosocial Research and Chief of Ambulatory Personality Disorder Services, McLean Hospital, Belmont, Massachusetts; Professor of Psychiatry, Harvard Medical School, Boston, Massachusetts

John M. Oldham, M.D.
Director, New York State Psychiatric Institute; Dollard Professor and Acting Chairman, Department of Psychiatry, Columbia University College of Physicians and Surgeons, New York, New York

J. Christopher Perry, M.P.H., M.D.
Professor of Psychiatry, McGill University; Director of Research, Institute of Community and Family Psychiatry, Sir Mortimer B. Davis–Jewish General Hospital, Montréal, Québec, Canada; Visiting Professor in Psychiatry, Harvard Medical School at The Austen Riggs Center, Stockbridge, Massachusetts

Michelle B. Riba, M.D.
Clinical Associate Professor of Psychiatry and Associate Chair for Education and Academic Affairs, Department of Psychiatry, University of Michigan Health System, Ann Arbor, Michigan

Michael H. Stone, M.D.

Professor of Clinical Psychiatry, Columbia University College of Physicians & Surgeons, New York, New York; Attending Psychiatrist, Mid-Hudson Forensic Psychiatric Hospital, New Hampton, New York

Peter Tyrer, M.D.

Professor of Community Psychiatry, Division of Neuroscience and Psychological Medicine, Imperial College School of Medicine, Paterson Centre, London, England

Introduction to the Review of Psychiatry Series

John M. Oldham, M.D.
Michelle B. Riba, M.D., Series Editors

2000 REVIEW OF PSYCHIATRY SERIES TITLES

- *Learning Disabilities: Implications for Psychiatric Treatment*
  EDITED BY LAURENCE L. GREENHILL, M.D.
- *Psychotherapy for Personality Disorders*
  EDITED BY JOHN G. GUNDERSON, M.D., AND GLEN O. GABBARD, M.D.
- *Ethnicity and Psychopharmacology*
  EDITED BY PEDRO RUIZ, M.D.
- *Complementary and Alternative Medicine and Psychiatry*
  EDITED BY PHILIP R. MUSKIN, M.D.
- *Pain: What Psychiatrists Need to Know*
  EDITED BY MARY JANE MASSIE, M.D.

The advances in knowledge in the field of psychiatry and the neurosciences in the last century can easily be described as breathtaking. As we embark on a new century and a new millennium, we felt that it would be appropriate for the 2000 Review of Psychiatry Series monographs to take stock of the state of that knowledge at the interface between normality and pathology. Although there may be nothing new under the sun, we are learning more about not-so-new things, such as how we grow and develop; who we are; how to differentiate between just being different from one another and being ill; how to recognize, treat, and perhaps prevent illness; how to identify our unique vulnerabilities; and how to deal with the inevitable stress and pain that await each of us.

In the early years of life, for example, how can we tell whether a particular child is just rowdier, less intelligent, or more adventuresome than another child—or is, instead, a child with a learning or behavior disorder? Clearly, the distinction is crucial, because newer and better treatments that now exist for early-onset disorders can smooth the path and enhance the chances for a solid future for children with such disorders. Yet, inappropriately labeling and treating a rambunctious but normal child can create problems rather than solve them. Greenhill and colleagues guide us through these waters, illustrating that a highly sophisticated methodology has been developed to make this distinction with accuracy, and that effective treatments and interventions are now at hand.

Once we have successfully navigated our way into early adulthood, we are supposed to have a pretty good idea (so the advice books say) of who we are. Of course, this stage of development does not come easy, nor at the same time, for all. Again, a challenge presents itself—that is, to differentiate between widely disparate varieties of temperament and character and when extremes of personality traits and styles should be recognized as disorders. And even when traits are so extreme that little dispute exists that a disorder is present, does that disorder represent who the person is, or is it something the individual either inherited or developed and might be able to overcome? In the fifth century B.C., Hippocrates described different personality types that he proposed were correlated with specific "body humors"; this ancient principle remains quite relevant, though the body humors of today are neurotransmitters. How low CNS serotonin levels need to be, for example, to produce disordered impulsivity is still being determined, yet new symptom-targeted treatment of such conditions with SSRIs is now well accepted. What has been at risk as the neurobiology of personality disorders has become increasingly understood is the continued recognition of the importance of psychosocial treatments for these disorders. Gunderson and Gabbard and their colleagues review the surprisingly robust evidence for the effectiveness of these approaches, including new uses and types of cognitive-behavioral and psychoeducational methods.

It is not just differences in personality that distinguish us from one another. Particularly in our new world of global communication and population migration, ethnic and cultural differences are more often part of life in our own neighborhoods than just exotic and unfamiliar aspects of faraway lands. Despite great strides overcoming fears and prejudices, much work remains to be done. At the same time, we must learn more about ways that we are different (not better or worse) genetically and biologically, because uninformed ignorance of these differences leads to unacceptable risks. Ruiz and colleagues carefully present what we now know and do not know about ethnicity and its effects on pharmacokinetics and pharmacodynamics.

An explosion of interest in and information about wellness—not just illness—surrounds us. How to achieve and sustain a healthy lifestyle, how to enhance successful aging, and how to benefit from "natural" remedies saturate the media. Ironically, although this seems to be a new phenomenon, the principles of complementary or alternative medicine are ancient. Some of our oldest and most widely used medications are derived from plants and herbs, and Eastern medicine has for centuries relied on concepts of harmony, relaxation, and meditation. Again, as the world shrinks, we are obligated to be open to ideas that may be new to us but not to others and to carefully evaluate their utility. Muskin and colleagues present a careful analysis of the most familiar and important components of complementary and alternative medicine, presenting a substantial database of information, along with tutorials on non-Western (hence nontraditional to us) concepts and beliefs.

Like it or not, life presents us with stress and pain. Pain management has not typically figured into mainstream psychiatric training or practice (with the exception of consultation-liaison psychiatry), yet it figures prominently in the lives of us all. Massie and colleagues provide us with a primer on what psychiatrists should know about the subject, and there is a great deal indeed that we should know.

Many other interfaces exist between psychiatry as a field of medicine, defining and treating psychiatric illnesses, and the rest of medicine—and between psychiatry and the many paths of the life cycle. These considerations are, we believe, among our top priorities as we begin the new millennium, and these volumes provide an in-depth review of some of the most important ones.

Foreword

John G. Gunderson, M.D.
Glen O. Gabbard, M.D.

The accounts of psychotherapy with patients who have personality disorders in this volume of the millennium edition of the Review of Psychiatry Series are timely, if not overdue. Efforts to review this topic were previously undertaken in the 1982, 1986, and 1992 volumes. In each case, the reviewers decried the lack of empirical work while underscoring its importance. The current review's timeliness is evident in the clinically instructive and empirically supported five chapters that follow. We presume that relatively few readers will have been aware of the significant advances in knowledge and sophistication unveiled in these chapters. The gradual rise of empirical bases for clinical practice marks a shift that can only grow. Still, the advances that have been made do little to diminish the public health significance of this topic.

About 13%–18% of the population have personality disorders (Weissman 1993; Zimmerman and Coryell 1989). The DSM-IV (American Psychiatric Association 1994) definition requiring significant subjective distress (like the mental state disorders in Axis I) or social impairment (for which the threshold for being "significant" seems in practice to be very high) combines with their expected long-term stability to make personality disorders a subject of enormous public health concern. Preliminary data from an ongoing collaborative study suggest that the amount of health care use and social impairment associated with having a personality disorder is very high and far exceeds that found in people with major depressive disorders who do not have a personality disorder (Bender et al., submitted). Against this background of high prevalence and high public health significance, the current review of psychotherapies indeed seems overdue.

A thoughtful review of three prior volumes in the Review of Psychiatry Series (1982, 1986, 1992), in which psychotherapies for personality disorders were the topic, and of the three editions of *Treatments of Psychiatric Disorders* (1989, 1995, in press) shows that although medications have a role, psychodynamic and, to a lesser extent, cognitive-behavioral therapies consistently have been the backbone of treatment plans recommended for personality disorders. Although differences exist in how responsive each type of personality disorder is expected to be to any psychotherapy (e.g., paranoid and antisocial personality disorders are not thought to be either motivated or responsive) and in how effective each type of psychotherapy is (e.g., cognitive-behavioral therapies are thought to be especially useful for avoidant and borderline personality disorders, whereas psychoanalysis may be the only effective treatment for narcissistic and obsessive-compulsive personality disorders), the general conclusion is that the major modality on which treatability rests is psychotherapy, with medications playing an adjunctive role.

Readers who are hoping to have empirically based guidelines for using psychotherapy for personality disorders will be disappointed. Although knowledge about treating borderline personality disorder is sufficient (notably, much of this is based on what *not* to do) to warrant the current American Psychiatric Association effort to develop official guidelines, many intermediary steps must be taken before psychotherapies, let alone the overall psychosocial treatment of personality disorders, can be prescribed with the specificity that manual-based therapies require. Certainly, the awareness of the complementary role of many modalities and of the need to judge "readiness" for psychotherapies is much better. Some patients with personality disorders may be ready for couples therapy or even medication before they will be ready for even a time-limited focused cognitive therapy, and maybe only then will they be motivated or able to undertake a longer-term dynamic therapy.

The definition of *psychotherapy* varies in these chapters. Perry and Bond's impressive and very encouraging review of effectiveness in Chapter 1 uses data from any and all nonpharmacological treatments. In Chapter 2, Gunderson discusses only one form of psychotherapy—individual psychodynamic (or psychoanalytic)—for one type of personality disorder—borderline. In Chapter

3, Gabbard, like Perry and Bond, uses a more generic definition of psychotherapy, but he is primarily concerned with conceptual issues and practical management to help clinicians in their efforts to combine medications with individual psychotherapies safely and effectively. In Chapter 4, Stone deals with a specific personality disorder—antisocial—and approaches treatment considerations from a broader perspective than psychotherapy. He suggests ways to determine which patients are treatable and which are not. Tyrer and Davidson, in Chapter 5, review the promising development of another specific type of psychotherapy (i.e., cognitive psychotherapies) but cover the application of this modality to all the personality disorders.

Clearly, these chapters cover only a small fraction of the issues that may be of value to clinicians. Some of these other issues are covered in the soon-to-be-published third edition of *Treatments of Psychiatric Disorders* (Gabbard, in press). Those reviews, like this one, leave readers with two firm conclusions. First, psychotherapies are essential, challenging, and rewarding for patients with personality disorders. Second, a gold mine of researchable questions are still awaiting answers, and their investigation also is essential, challenging, and potentially very rewarding.

References

American Psychiatric Association: Diagnostic and Statistical Manual of Mental Disorders, 4th Edition. Washington, DC, American Psychiatric Association, 1994

Bender DS, Dolan RT, Skodol AE, et al: Treatment utilization by patients with personality disorders (submitted)

Gabbard GO (ed): Treatments of Psychiatric Disorders, 3rd Edition. Washington, DC, American Psychiatric Association (in press)

Weissman MM: The epidemiology of personality disorders: a 1990 update. J Personal Disord 7 (suppl):44–62, 1993

Zimmerman M, Coryell W: DSM-III personality disorder diagnoses in a nonpatient sample: demographic correlates and comorbidity. Arch Gen Psychiatry 46:682–689, 1989

Chapter 1

Empirical Studies of Psychotherapy for Personality Disorders

J. Christopher Perry, M.P.H., M.D.
Michael Bond, M.D.

Most research on personality disorders has emphasized diagnostic issues and the persistent problems with interpersonal and social functioning over time. Similarly, the clinical literature has emphasized the difficulties in management and treatment, often suggesting modifications in technique to improve clinical outcomes. As suggested two decades ago (Vaillant and Perry 1980), many still view the personality disorders as the stepchildren of psychiatry because they lack the knowledge that these disorders can improve with psychotherapy. This review of empirical studies of psychotherapy for the personality disorders suggests that the view that the personality disorders are intractable to treatment is due for a major revision. We review the relevant outcome and related studies of psychotherapy process and then summarize major and suggestive findings, with their clinical implications for psychotherapy.

As with other reviews, this review stands on the shoulders of previous reviews, including Perry et al. 1999; Reich and Vasile 1993; Roth and Fonagy 1996; Sanislow and McGlashan 1998; Shea 1993; and Target 1998. Specific coverage of the individual personality disorder types also can be found in chapter reviews of individual personality disorders in *Treatments of Psychiatric Disorders*, 3rd Edition (Gabbard, in press). The current review differs from earlier reviews by including the most recent empirical literature and striving to fit their findings into a common framework, rather than proceeding as a detailed, perhaps confusing, review of their disparate designs and findings. The result should facilitate drawing conclusions across studies. We examine evidence for the clinical effectiveness, efficacy, degree of improvement, differential effects of diagnosis, proportion of patients who remit, and proportion who drop out of psychotherapy. We then consider some important process variables, especially the therapeutic alliance and therapist interventions, before summarizing our conclusions.

Effectiveness of Psychotherapy for Personality Disorders

Finding Common Approaches to Comparing Studies

Scientific studies usually report the significance of their findings with probability statistics, but these alone do not indicate *how much* change occurred following active treatment. The fact that the treatments offered, the study designs, and the samples are not comparable further complicates the effort to summarize what is known about psychotherapy for personality disorders.

We have taken three approaches to this problem. The first and most inclusive approach is to make a box score that includes a few study characteristics and the study's findings of whether the sample improved significantly.

The second approach is to calculate a within-condition effect size for each of the measures used in a study, which yields a pure number representing how many standard deviations the sample has changed on a given measure from intake. Because most studies use multiple measures, each study is represented by the mean of each measure's effect size. Thus, the same metric can be used to compare across measures and studies. To calculate this within-condition effect size for a measure, the pretreatment score is subtracted from the posttreatment score and then divided by the standard deviation of the measure at intake. This approach measures how much change has occurred but can be used only for those studies reporting all three descriptive statistics (mean at intake and its standard deviation, mean at outcome). Studies that fail to do so can be used only in the box score approach.

The third approach can be used for studies that report the percentage of subjects who no longer have symptoms that meet full criteria for a personality disorder at termination or follow-up. Remission or recovery from full personality disorder criteria still may be associated with some remaining personality disorder traits. This third approach is therefore not fully analogous to remission of an episodic disorder, such as major depression, in which the definition of remission requires no or minimal symptoms remaining. We present findings of all three approaches as the data allow.

Is Psychotherapy Associated With Significant Improvement?

Table 1–1 displays some of the characteristics and findings of the studies of psychotherapy for personality disorders. We found 22 studies with at least one treatment arm for personality disorders that reported the outcome of psychotherapy with some generally accepted measures. One study (Piper et al. 1993) combined personality disorder and depressed patients in the results but is included because more than two-thirds had a personality disorder. Five studies made some comparison with non–personality disorder groups also treated (Diguer et al. 1993; Fahy et al. 1993; Karterud et al. 1992; Patience et al. 1995; Wilberg et al. 1998). Four were outpatient controlled trials with random assignment to active treatment or control condition (wait-list or treatment as usual), and one-fifth had a no-treatment condition but without random assignment (Alden 1989; Piper et al. 1993; Shea et al. 1990; A. Winston et al. 1994). Most studies used individual psychotherapy, whereas one used a short-term (Liberman and Eckman 1981) and one used a long-term (Dolan et al. 1997) inpatient program, two used residential programs (Hafner and Holme 1996; Krawitz 1997), and three used day treatment (Karterud et al. 1992; Piper et al. 1993; Wilberg et al. 1998). All studies reported some significant, positive changes in personality disorder groups following active psychotherapy.

Table 1–1. Description of studies and summary of effect sizes (ESs)

Study	Diagnosis (N)	Duration	Follow-up	Dropout	Treatment	Self-report ES	Observer-rated ES	% Recovered
Liberman and Eckman 1981[a]	BPD (24)	10 days	9 months	17%	BT	1.27	0.93	
Woody et al. 1985[a]	Total (110) Therapy (n = 62) O only O + depression O + depression + ASP O + ASP only	6 months	1 month	NR	CBT and dynamic		0.39 0.53 0.50 0.18	
Alden 1989[a]	AVPD (76)	10 weeks	3 months	5%	CBT Control	0.91 0.13	0.80 0.19	
Shea et al. 1990	MDE (239) PDs Cluster A (47) B (40) C (155)	16 weeks	—	All PDs: 31% A 36% B 40% C 28%	CBT IPT Imipramine Placebo + CM	Improved: PDs similar to non-PDs; Cluster A less		PDs improved but had lower percentage of MDE recovered and poorer social and leisure outcome
Stevenson and Meares 1992[a]	BPD (30)	12 months	1 year	27%	Dynamic	0.94	0.95	30%

Table 1–1. Description of studies and summary of effect sizes (ESs) *(continued)*

Study	Diagnosis (N)	Duration	Follow-up	Dropout	Treatment	Self-report ES	Observer-rated ES	% Recovered
Karterud et al. 1992[a]	Total (97) SPD (13) BPD (34) Other PD (26) No PD (23)	6 months	At end of therapy	24%	Dynamic No PD All PDs SPD BPD Other PDs	1.36 0.82 0.66 1.02 0.78	1.48 0.46 −0.03 0.45 0.96	
Fahy et al. 1993[a]	Total (39) PDs (14)	8 weeks	6.8 months	8%	CBT: PDs No PDs	1.33 2.47		
Hoglend 1993[a]	Total (45) PDs (15)	Mean 27.5 Weekly sessions: brief = 18; medium = 42	4 years	Total 16% PD: 33% No PD: 7%	Dynamic Brief Medium		2.51 (1.99) (2.57)	40%

Table 1–1. Description of studies and summary of effect sizes (ESs) (*continued*)

Study	Diagnosis (N)	Duration	Follow-up	Dropout	Treatment	Self-report ES	Observer-rated ES	% Recovered
Diguer et al. 1993[a]	Total (25) PD + MDE (12) MDE only (13)	16 weeks	6 months	0%	Dynamic PD + MDE MDE only	1.67 2.77	2.41 3.56	
Piper et al. 1993[b]	Total (120) Depressed (85) PDs (72): DPD, BPD	18 weeks × 5 days/week = 90 session days	1 year: 8 months after termination	Total: 38% Group: 42% Wait-list: 32%	Day treatment Dynamic groups Wait-list	0.80 0.17	1.27 0.14	
A. Winston et al. 1994[a]	Cluster C PDs (81)	40 weeks	1.5 years	15%	Dynamic BAP STAP Wait-list	1.20 1.35 0.45		
Linehan et al. 1994[a]	BPD (26)	12 months		19%	CBT-DBT Treatment as usual	0.82 0.18	1.20 0.81	
Monsen et al. 1995[a]	Total (25) PDs (23)	25.4 months	5.2 years	16%	Dynamic	0.92	2.30	68%
Munroe-Blum and Marziali 1995[a]	BPD (110) Entered treatment (79)	Group: 35 weeks Individual: unspecified	2 years	Group: 42% Individual: 37%	Group IGP or Dynamic individual	Combined total: 1.10	Combined total: 0.67	

Table 1–1. Description of studies and summary of effect sizes (ESs) *(continued)*

Study	Diagnosis (N)	Duration	Follow-up	Dropout	Treatment	Self-report ES	Observer-rated ES	% Recovered
Patience et al. 1995	MDE (113) MDE only (63) PD + MDE (37)	16 weeks	1.5 years	7% overall	CBT Social work GP Drug: AMI		All four treatments equivalent; acute recovery of MDE	PDs: 47% No PD: 67%
Budman et al. 1996[a]	Total (48) Cluster B, C (24)	78 weeks 72 sessions	None	51%	Interpersonal group		0.84	69%
Hafner and Holme 1996	PDs (48) BPD (34)	64 days × 5 days/week	6 months	Not reported	Residential: interpersonal groups	GSI and hostility decreased	Significantly fewer days in hospital: prior vs. subsequent year	
Krawitz 1997	PDs (31) Cluster C (25) BPD (6)	17 weeks in residence × 4 days/week = 68 session-days	2 years	3%	Semiresidential: dynamic groups	2.33	1.66	

Table 1–1. Description of studies and summary of effect sizes (ESs) *(continued)*

Study	Diagnosis (N)	Duration	Follow-up	Dropout	Treatment	Self-report ES	Observer-rated ES	% Recovered
Dolan et al. 1997	Severe PDs Treated (70) Untreated (67)	7 months in residence × 5 days/ week = 150 session-days	1 year	NR	Inpatient therapeutic community groups vs. untreated	1.43 0.64		
Barber 1997	PDs (35) AVPD (23) OCPD (12)	Up to 52 weekly sessions 34.9 AVPD 50.1 OCPD	—	AVPD 46% OPCD 7%	Individual Dynamic	1.00 total AVPD 0.98 OCPD 1.05	1.30 total AVPD 1.37 OCPD 1.16	62% 85%
Wilberg et al. 1998	Poorly function-ing patients (183) PDs (159)	18 weeks × 5 days/week = 90 session-days	—	22%	Day treatment: dynamic and CBT groups	No PDs: 0.82 All PDs: 0.54 Cluster A: 0.84 B: 0.45 C: 0.60 PD NOS: 0.30	2.46 1.45 Cluster A: 0.93 B: 1.44 C: 1.50 PD NOS: 1.60	

Table 1-1. Description of studies and summary of effect sizes (ESs) (*continued*)

Study	Diagnosis (N)	Duration	Follow-up	Dropout	Treatment	Self-report ES	Observer-rated ES	% Recovered
Rosenthal et al. 1999	PDs (20) All Cluster C PDs	40 weeks	1.3 years (6 months posttreatment)	40%	Brief supportive psychotherapy	0.80		
Summary								
Active psychotherapies for non-PDs	**Mean ES** (Median, n = number of treatment arms)						**1.85 ± 0.92** (1.92, n = 4)	**1.68 ± 1.34** (1.48, n = 5)
Active psychotherapies for PD groups	**Mean ES** (Median, n = number of treatment arms)						**1.14 ± 0.41** (1.02, n = 18)	**1.32 ± 0.68** (1.20, n = 17)
Wait-list or treatment as usual	**Mean ES** (Median, n = number of treatment arms)						**0.31 ± 0.22** (0.18, n = 5)	**0.38 ± 0.37** (0.19, n = 3)

Abbreviations (alphabetically): AMI = amitriptyline; ASP = antisocial PD; AVPD = avoidant PD; BAP = brief adaptive therapy; BPD = borderline PD; BT = behavior therapy; CBT = cognitive-behavioral therapy; CM = clinical management; DBT = dialectical behavior therapy; DPD = dependent personality disorder; GP = general practitioner; GSI = General Severity Index of the Brief Symptom Inventory; IGP = interpersonal group psychotherapy; IPT = interpersonal psychotherapy; MDE = major depressive episode; NOS = not otherwise specified; NR = not reported; O = opiate dependence; OCPD = obsessive-compulsive personality disorder; PD = personality disorder; SPD = schizotypal PD; STAP = short-term anxiety provoking therapy.

[a]Studies reported in Perry et al. 1999.
[b]Effect size data supplied to authors by Dr. Piper (1996).
[c]n = number of treatment arms.

Effect Size of Psychotherapy for Personality Disorders

The second approach examines those studies whose results can be compared with a common metric. Perry et al. (1999) used within-condition effect sizes to examine change in self-report and observer-rated measures in 15 studies of active psychotherapy. These were examined separately because of the likelihood that self-report ratings (e.g., target complaints, Beck Depression Inventory [BDI]) might differ from observer-rated measures (e.g., Global Assessment Scale). The mean effect size for improvement in self-report measures was 1.11 (median 1.02), and it was 1.29 (median 0.94) for observer-rated measures, with both means significantly greater than zero ($P = 0.0001$ and 0.0002, respectively). This represents a large degree of improvement. By contrast, improvement among those in wait-list or treatment-as-usual control conditions yielded lower mean effect sizes for self-report (mean 0.25, median 0.18 in three studies) and for observer-rated (mean 0.50, median 0.50 in two studies) outcomes. These latter effect sizes represent only small to medium degrees of improvement.

Table 1–1 also updates the above findings with an additional five studies for which some effect sizes were calculable (Barber 1997; Dolan et al. 1997; Krawitz 1997; Piper et al. 1993; Wilberg et al. 1998). The mean and median effect sizes for self-report and observer-rated outcomes (see last row of Table 1–1) are greater than 1.0, similar but slightly higher than the earlier published figures noted above, and also highly significantly greater than zero (both $P < 0.0001$).

Efficacy of Psychotherapy

Randomized, controlled treatment trials provide the strongest evidence of the efficacy of psychotherapy for personality disorders. These trials allow treatment effects to be examined after taking into account improvement due to regression to the mean associated with the control condition. In a review, Perry and colleagues (1999) found three psychotherapy studies that compared an active therapy with a wait-list or nonspecific control condition for individuals with avoidant (Alden 1989), parasuicidal borderline

(Linehan et al. 1994), or largely Cluster C personality disorder types (A. Winston et al. 1994). Among the three randomized, controlled trials, the within-condition effect size of the control condition was subtracted from that of the active psychotherapy; a positive number reflected the psychotherapy advantage. For self-report measures, the unweighted mean difference was 0.75, which was significantly greater than zero ($P = 0.006$), or a mean of 0.78 when weighted by sample size ($P = 0.002$), indicating about three-quarters of a standard deviation more improvement for the psychotherapies. This is a moderate to large difference.

In the two studies reporting observer-rated measures, the differences in effect size yielded an unweighted mean difference of 0.50 ($P = 0.14$) and a mean difference of 0.57 ($P = 0.085$) when weighted by sample size. If one includes the Piper et al. (1993) study, which included some depressed patients without a personality disorder, the mean observer-rated difference increases to 0.71 unweighted ($n = 3$, $t = 3.23$, $P = 0.08$) or 0.84 weighted by the number of completers ($n = 3$, $t = 4.21$, $P = 0.052$). These differences represent about one-half to three-quarters of a standard deviation more improvement for active psychotherapy over control subjects, but more studies are required to determine whether this finding will become stable and significant. Overall, the evidence for the efficacy of psychotherapy is strong for self-report measures and suggestive for observer-rated measures. Nonetheless, the small number of studies warrants caution.

Differential Effects by Diagnosis

In all studies with both personality disorder and non–personality disorder patients, the group with personality disorders did not improve to the same degree as the group without personality disorders (Diguer et al. 1993; Fahy et al. 1993; Hardy et al. 1995; Karterud et al. 1992; Woody et al. 1985). Table 1–1 summarizes these studies at the bottom, indicating larger, substantial mean effect sizes for non–personality disorder groups (self-report 1.85, observer-rated 1.68). The National Institute of Mental Health Treatment of Depression Collaborative Research Project (Shea et al. 1990) obtained a similar finding for some measures, most notably, a lower percentage of recovery from depression and poorer social functioning at termination among those with a personality disorder.

Karterud et al. (1992) examined specific personality disorder types and found that patients with Cluster C personality disorders improved more than borderline personality disorder patients who, in turn, improved more than schizotypal personality disorder patients. Schizotypal personality disorder appeared to require a longer treatment than the 7 months allotted. In his own case series, Stone (1983) also noted that patients with schizotypal personality disorder showed more limited improvements than patients with borderline personality disorder. Similarly, Woody et al. (1985) found that patients with antisocial personality disorder did not have good outcomes except when depression was comorbid. The association with depression may indicate the ability to form attachments and develop a positive therapeutic alliance (Gerstley et al. 1989).

What Changes With Psychotherapy?

Table 1–2 displays the mean effect sizes for any measure used in at least two psychotherapy studies. Fourteen studies (15 treatment arms) allowed the calculation of within-condition effect sizes for six measures. Four measures yielded mean effect sizes greater than 1, which could be considered a large degree of change. Improvement in target complaints showed the largest effect. This is understandable, as the initial complaints leading one to seek therapy may be somewhat more changeable than the underlying problems because the former are influenced by initially high levels of distress that diminish early on, whereas the latter change more slowly. Improvement in depressive symptoms by the self-report BDI had the next largest effect. Because the personality disorder patients in two studies that used the BDI had a major depressive episode (Diguer et al. 1993; Hardy et al. 1995), this finding should be most relevant to patients with personality disorders who are depressed, yet findings were comparable in two groups of personality disorder patients not selected for depression (Barber 1997). Perhaps the latter represent improvement in distress and depressive-like cognitions and experiences. Global functioning, by either the Global Assessment Scale or the Health-

Table 1–2. Effect sizes for specific measures used in at least two studies

Study	Target complaints	BDI	GAS or HSRS	General symptoms	IIP	Social adjustment
Alden 1989	1.31					
Karterud et al. 1992			0.46	0.82		
Stevenson and Meares 1992				0.94		
Diguer et al. 1993		1.67	2.41			
Piper et al. 1993				1.17		0.64
A. Winston et al. 1994	2.28			0.70		0.86
Hogland 1993			2.51			
Linehan et al. 1994			1.36	1.00		1.07
Munroe-Blum and Marziali 1995						0.49
Hardy et al. 1995		1.84		1.24	1.53	
Krawitz 1997			1.66	2.33		
Barber 1997						
AVPD		1.32			0.88	
OCPD		2.21			0.41	
Wilberg et al. 1998			1.45	0.55	0.52	
Rosenthal et al. 1999					0.52	
Mean effect size	**1.80**	**1.79**	**1.64**	**1.10**	**0.77**	**0.77**
±SD	.48	.45	.76	.55	.46	.25

Note. AVPD = avoidant personality disorder; BDI = Beck Depression Inventory; GAS = Global Assessment Scale; HSRS = Health-Sickness Rating Scale; IIP = Inventory of Interpersonal Problems; OCPD = obsessive-compulsive personality disorder.

Sickness Rating Scale, was close to depressive symptoms in effect size. The fourth largest effect size was found for general self-report symptoms, measured by instruments such as the Symptom Checklist–90 (SCL-90). The two measures with effect sizes less than 1.0 were those most directly reflecting personality functioning: interpersonal functioning, as measured by the self-report Inventory of Interpersonal Problems (IIP), and social role functioning. This fits with the clinical observation that social functioning and basic personality disorder traits themselves improve more slowly than symptoms. Unfortunately, the above studies and measures do not directly address the degree to which core psychopathology and the underlying mechanisms of personality functioning change with treatment. A generation of studies that examine the role of theoretically selected mechanisms are required to redress this.

Treatment Length and Remission From Full Personality Disorder Criteria

Perry et al. (1999) examined four studies that assessed their treated patients for personality disorder criteria at follow-up (Budman et al. 1996; Hoglend 1993; Monsen et al. 1995; Stevenson and Meares 1992). The studies used dynamic-interpersonal therapies, ranging from a mean of 27.5 weeks to 25.4 months, including both individual and group modalities in once- or twice-weekly sessions. The diagnostic mix included Cluster B and C disorders, but 53% of the patients had borderline personality disorder. After a mean of 78 sessions over a mean of 67 weeks (1.3 years), the mean proportion remitted was 52% (95% confidence interval 13.1%–90.4%), which differed significantly from zero ($P = 0.01$). Perry et al. (1999) used simple linear regression methods to create a model from these data and compared it with a published model of remission of borderline personality disorder from natural history studies (Perry 1993). The active therapy model was not statistically significant, but it is useful for heuristic purposes. The active therapy model estimated that 25.8% of personality disorder cases remitted per year of therapy, a rate sevenfold larger than the natural history of borderline personality disorder (3.7% remitted per year, with remission of 50% of cases requiring 10.5 years of naturalistic follow-up). Because the range of studies used in either model only went up to about 70% of the subjects remitted, neither model should be extrapolated beyond that. An important constraint is that the studies done with both models included only people who remained in the studies (completers), omitting those who dropped out. The more rigorous intent-to-treat remission figures are likely to be lower and are unknown as of yet.

Barber (1997) also reported a study of patients with avoidant and obsessive-compulsive personality disorders treated with up to 52 sessions of dynamic psychotherapy. At study termination, 61% and 85% of the patients recovered, respectively. Figure 1–1 compares the percentage recovered in the five natural history studies of borderline personality disorder, discussed earlier in this chapter, and the percentage recovered in the active psychotherapy studies (the four noted earlier plus two treatment arms from Barber 1997). These six active treatment arms were conducted over a mean of 1.24 years, and the mean percentage recovered was 58.8% ± 20.3%, or 54.4% when weighted by the number completing treatment (similar to the above). However, as shown in Figure 1–1, differences were found between the treatment results with predominantly Cluster C patients (mostly dependent, avoidant, obsessive-compulsive) and those with predominantly Clusters B and A (mostly borderline personality disorder) patients.

We repeated the simple linear regression models used above but considered the predominantly Cluster B and C samples separately. The Cluster C treatments yielded a weighted mean of 60.9% recovered after a mean of 37.5 sessions over a mean duration of almost 1 year (0.96 years). By contrast, the Cluster B treatments yielded a weighted mean of 50.4% recovered after a mean of 94.7 sessions over a mean duration of 1.52 years. The rate of recovery from the model of the three Cluster C treatments was 52.0% per year or 1.9% per session, whereas in the three Cluster B treatments, the rate of recovery was 36.2% per year or 0.33% per session. The contrasting results when Cluster B predominates over Cluster C are further exemplified by the ratio of their percentage recovered per session: B:C = 1.9%:0.33%, or 5.9. Without being able to control for sources of measurement error and other factors that might influence the recovery rates, this ratio suggests that Cluster B pa-

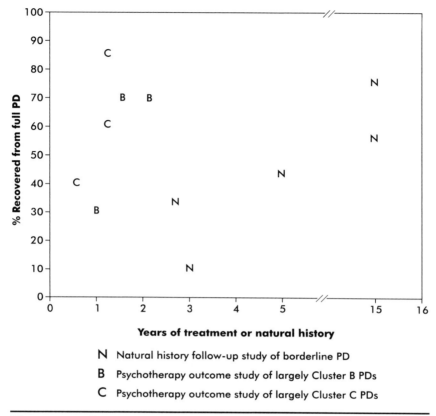

Figure 1–1. Percentage recovered from full personality disorder (PD) criteria by years of treatment or natural history in three groups of studies.

tients, principally those with borderline personality disorder, will take about six sessions for every one session required for a Cluster C patient for a comparable effect on recovery. The small number of treatment arms, three each, precludes determining whether these models and differences between the Clusters are statistically significant. In addition, based on the few studies, the results are likely to be somewhat unstable, and their generalizability to other samples has yet to be determined. They should not, therefore, be accepted as valid and must be interpreted with great caution. This is especially true for their use as a basis to determine a priori how many sessions a patient with a given diagnosis should require to recover from full personality disorder criteria. Nonetheless, these findings descriptively represent our current level of empirical knowledge about recovery.

In summary, for Cluster B and C personality disorders, remaining in therapy may be associated with a remission rate up to sevenfold faster than the natural remission rate for borderline personality disorder. Furthermore, Cluster C patients appear to recover in fewer sessions over less time than Cluster B patients. However, additional studies are required to validate what are now considered intriguing hypotheses.

Diagnosis, Treatment Type and Duration, and Measurement Perspective

Perry and colleagues (1999) examined improvement effect sizes by treatment duration and measurement perspective. In examining self-report measures, the mean self-report effect sizes of the five shorter-term therapies (16 weeks or less) were significantly larger than those of the seven longer-term studies (1.38 vs. 0.92, $P = 0.02$). This raised the question of whether self-report measures reflect some transient change, a so-called honeymoon effect that diminishes somewhat in longer treatments. This was not found with observer-rated measures. Unfortunately, in the existing studies, treatment type and duration were confounded with diagnoses. Cluster C disorders generally were given shorter-duration treatments, usually cognitive-behavioral therapy (CBT), whereas borderline and other more severe personality disorder types tended to receive longer treatments, usually dynamic therapy. The one longer-term CBT for parasuicidal borderline personality disorder patients (Linehan et al. 1994) had one of the lowest self-report effect sizes, which could reflect diagnosis or treatment type or duration. However, at the same time, it showed a mean observer-rated effect size near the mean of 15 studies, which included significant decreases in suicide attempts. This highlights the caution required in comparing results from self-report and observer-rated measurement perspectives. We need to understand better the factors associated with divergence or convergence in the report of feeling better (self-report) and the observation that one is actually doing better.

This paradoxical self-report phenomenon must be considered when comparing treatment effects, lest one mistakenly assume a shorter-term treatment is better than a longer-term treatment, when other patient, measurement, or treatment factors may be responsible for differences in effect sizes. Three possible explanations should be considered. First, most shorter-duration studies are aimed at treating less severe disturbances (e.g., from Cluster C); these patients may then report feeling better to a greater degree than more disturbed patients would who are receiving longer-term therapy. Second, longer-duration studies may be more often targeted toward borderline and other more severe personality disorder types, who might not report as much subjective improvement as Cluster C patients, regardless of treatment duration. The findings of Linehan et al. (1994) are consistent with this theory. Third, self-reported improvement may be initially highly responsive to treatment in the short term (honeymoon effect) but then may diminish somewhat as longer-term therapeutic work continues, whereas observer-rated improvement may be more tied to duration of treatment. This is consistent with findings from a more heterogeneous sample that measures of self-report distress and character have different patterns of response over a year of psychotherapy (Kopta et al. 1994). Use of both measurement perspectives, not just self-report, with long-term follow-up should mitigate against this potential bias favoring shorter-term therapies.

Dropouts From Psychotherapy

Earlier studies have shown that dropout from psychotherapy is a substantial problem, especially in borderline personality disorder (Gunderson et al. 1989; Skodol et al. 1983), even when treatment is generally seen as successful (Waldinger and Gunderson 1984). Perry et al. (1999) found that a mean of 21.8% ± 14.7% (range 0%–51%) of patients dropped out from 14 active psychotherapy studies. This rate compares favorably with the National Institute of Mental Health Treatment of Depression Collaborative Research Program, which had a 31% dropout rate for personality disorders across all treatments, with the most among Clusters B (40%) and A (36%) and the least for Cluster C (28%) (Shea et al. 1990). The expanded list of studies in Table 1–1 produced a similar mean proportion of treatment dropouts (22.4% ± 15.5%).

Perry et al. (1999) found two treatment predictors of dropout. First, the two longer-term group therapy conditions (Budman et al. 1996; Munroe-Blum and Marziali 1995) had the highest percentage of dropouts (42% and 51%, respectively). Munroe-Blum and Marziali (1995) further noted that many of their patients with borderline personality disorder dropped out on learning that they were randomized to group therapy, even before the therapy began! Budman et al. (1996) noted that borderline personality disorder patients were particularly likely to drop out of group therapy and recommended adding individual treatment to group therapy, as Linehan et al. (1994) have done. These observations raise concerns, given the popularity of the group modality as a response to treatment costs. If limiting the choice of therapies to a group modality alone results in a high proportion of treatment refusal, especially among those with borderline personality disorder, then clinical settings may be excluding patients needing treatment.

Second, treatments of shorter duration (less than 16 weeks) had a mean lower percentage of dropouts than those of longer duration (8.2% vs. 29.3%, $P = 0.004$). The mean dropout rate for longer-duration treatment studies is comparable to the mean dropout rate of 28% for the natural history follow-up studies of borderline personality disorder (Perry 1993). This finding might be expected, because the longer the treatment, the greater the opportunity to drop out. However, other factors such as specific personality disorder type and treatment type also may influence dropping out (e.g., shorter-term treatments tended to include healthier Cluster C patients in CBT). Nevertheless, any new therapy being tested or any clinician or agency offering long- or short-term psychotherapy for personality disorders can use these dropout figures as a benchmark against which to compare themselves and improve on.

A third factor may operate in some cases to limit dropout: having nowhere else to go. For example, Krawitz (1997) reported that only one patient (3%) dropped out from a semiresidential program. Although the description of the program appears intriguingly attractive from a potential patient's point of view, the program resides in a largely rural setting, which also may limit competing treatment options. This factor may be difficult to ascertain, but the converse is certainly worth considering. Any treatment program in an area with limited alternative treatment options that has a high proportion of dropouts should consider that it has a serious problem requiring attention.

Other Factors Associated With Dropping Out

Individuals with personality disorders have interpersonal difficulties that may carry over into psychotherapy and affect the development of a therapeutic alliance. A deteriorating or poor therapeutic alliance may then lead to premature treatment termination. Gunderson et al. (1989) examined early discontinuance from psychotherapy among 60 newly hospitalized borderline personality disorder patients. Over 6 months of follow-up, 36 (60%) discontinued therapy. The most common cause (26 [72%] of those dropping out) was covert opposition, familial resistance, or angry dissatisfaction with treatment. Interestingly, those dropping out were healthier on some measures than those remaining in therapy.

Samsone et al. (1991) examined the treatment impressions and termination experiences of faculty clinicians who treated borderline personality disorder. The most commonly reported reasons for termination were that 1) the patient did not see the purpose of treatment or 2) the patient terminated through acting-out behaviors. A slight majority of clinicians reported that they had cured at least some of the borderline personality disorders.

Hilsenroth et al. (1998) explored the ability of specific DSM-IV (American Psychiatric Association 1994) Cluster B personality disorder criteria to predict continuance in supportive-expressive, insight-oriented psychotherapy. Five criteria predicted 31% of the variance. Three criteria predicted continuation: borderline personality disorder criterion 1: "frantic efforts to avoid real or imagined abandonment" (p. 654); borderline personality disorder criterion 8: "inappropriate, intense anger or difficulty controlling anger" (p. 654); and histrionic personality disorder criterion 8: "considers relationships to be more intimate than they actually are" (p. 658). Two criteria predicted premature termination:

narcissistic personality disorder criterion 4: "requires excessive admiration" (p. 661); and antisocial personality disorder criterion 7: "lack of remorse, as indicated by being indifferent to or rationalizing having hurt, mistreated, or stolen from another" (p. 650). These findings suggest that the ability or need for attachment and affective availability predicted continuation, whereas self-absorption and indifference to others predicted termination. The identification of these and other patient factors should prove helpful as future research connects which treatments can most likely retain which patients.

Overall, patient factors appear important in predicting retention or premature termination, but much more extensive exploration of these factors is required. Any specific psychotherapy will need to address how to deal with patients who present with or develop risk factors for premature termination.

Findings From Psychotherapy Process Research

The Therapeutic Alliance

One of the most robust areas of research in psychotherapy is the importance of a positive therapeutic alliance as a predictor of good outcome. In general, the alliance established early in therapy is particularly predictive of outcome, more than later alliance or the average across treatment (Horvath and Luborsky 1993). It was surprising that in the National Institute of Mental Health Treatment of Depression Collaborative Research Project the patient's alliance predicted more of the outcome variance across all treatment conditions, including placebo and clinical management, than the type of treatment the patient received (Krupnick et al. 1996).

Patients' characteristics, especially core psychiatric disorders and level of disturbance, appear to influence the development of the alliance. Gerstley et al. (1989) found that the ability to form a positive alliance was a crucial factor for a subset of opiate-dependent patients with antisocial personality disorder who had a favorable response to psychotherapy. Coupled with that study's previous finding—that only the antisocial personality disorder patients with comorbid depression had a good outcome (Woody et al. 1985)—it appears that the presence of depression may indicate the ability to form attachments and to develop a positive therapeutic alliance, which predicted better outcomes. Piper and colleagues (1991) reported that quality of object relations may influence the level of therapeutic alliance and outcome. Yoemans et al. (1994) found that a positive alliance as well as patient severity predicted dropout in long-term therapy for borderline disorder. In a study of group therapy for patients with borderline personality disorder, Marziali et al. (1997) found that the patients' ratings of alliance to the group were significant predictors of outcome, even more so than ratings of the degree of group cohesiveness.

The pattern of change in early alliance appears to be predictive of outcome, as first noted by Foreman and Marmar (1985). In a sample of mostly patients with a personality disorder, Piper et al. (1995) found that among patients with low quality of object relations, the change pattern (slope) of the alliance was a more significant predictor than the overall level of the alliance, although both made unique contributions to change, whereas in patients with high quality of object relations, no significant variation in slopes occurred, so the overall level of the alliance was a better predictor. Thus, in the early phase of therapy for personality disorders, therapists should monitor changes in the alliance carefully, addressing concerns about the alliance when it deteriorates or fails to improve.

Recent therapy manuals have emphasized the importance of addressing ruptures in the alliance as soon as they occur to facilitate both retention and positive work. This is demonstrated by the similarities between two different theoretical treatment approaches for borderline personality disorder when comparing the thematic priorities they direct a therapist to follow in a given session. In Linehan's (1993) CBT approach of dialectical behavior therapy, the first priority is to decrease suicidal behaviors, but the second priority is to decrease therapy-interfering behaviors. From a psychodynamic point of view, Kernberg et al. (1991) specified a similar first priority, attending to suicidal and homocidal threats, followed by four priorities addressing breaches in the therapeutic alliance: attending to 1) overt threats to treatment continuity, 2) dishonesty or deliberate withholding in sessions, 3) contract breaches, and 4) in-session acting out. This similarity is an important example in which a robust finding in the research literature, which converges with clinical observation, has informed the treatment manuals.

Research on Therapists' Interventions

Support Versus Exploration

There is a burgeoning interest in studying the differential relationship between therapists' interventions and patient outcomes. One commonly emerging way to divide therapists' interventions is the dichotomy between supportive and exploratory or interpretive interventions (Bond et al. 1998). Supportive interventions include reflection, clarification, and the offering of emotional support, encouragement, and concrete advice. Exploratory, expressive, or interpretive interventions include the exploration and interpretation of the patient's defenses, patterns of relating to others (object relations), and, specifically, transference in the therapy. Confrontation, a specialized form of directly interpreting defensive or transference phenomena, also is considered exploratory or expressive (Gabbard et al. 1994). However, the available research yields only a foreshadowing of what could constitute an empirical basis for the conduct of successful therapy with personality disorders. In a summary of the results of the Menninger study of psychotherapy and psychoanalysis in disturbed patients, many with personality disorders, Wallerstein (1989) concluded that both supportive and interpretive interventions are often mixed together, and both can lead to structural change, that is, improvement in the basic underlying personality structure.

Gabbard et al. (1994) examined the effect of different types of interventions on the alliance in three borderline patients whose therapies were audiotaped. These investigators found that transference interpretations were "high-risk, high-gain," concluding that they must be offered along with supportive interventions in the presence of a strong therapeutic alliance. Transference interpretations in the context of a weak alliance risk a rapid deterioration in the alliance. In a study of five borderline patients, Bond et al. (1998) found that whenever the alliance was already weak transference interpretations were followed by a deterioration in the therapeutic alliance, whereas whenever the alliance was solid, the interpretations were followed by enhanced working. Among patients with either a weak or a strong alliance, supportive interventions and defense interpretations enhanced therapeutic work without increasing defensiveness. Furthermore, supportive interventions seemed to prepare the way for repair of ruptures in the alliance and exploration.

Focal Adherence Versus Less Structured Exploration

The briefer psychotherapies are usually characterized by attempts to maintain a focus on the patient's main issues or dynamics. Hoglend and Piper (1995) examined the degree to which the therapist maintained a dynamic focus in two patient samples given brief psychotherapies. In both samples, high focal adherence was modestly associated with good outcome in patients with high quality of object relations. By contrast, high focal adherence was associated with poorer outcome among those with lower quality of object relations, often associated with a personality disorder diagnosis. The authors suggested that the latter group of patients may resist the therapist's focus on one dynamic theme, experiencing him or her as critical, rejecting, or dominating. Furthermore, "patients who are more dependent and who probably struggle with problems of trust, often require unfocused listening and more flexible interventions from the therapist" (Hoglend and Piper 1995, p. 626). This may be a significant factor limiting the effectiveness of briefer therapies for personality disorders.

Insight and Affect

A. Winston et al. (1994) tested two forms of psychotherapy in a group of patients with largely Cluster C personality disorders. Short-term dynamic psychotherapy focuses directly on the patient's defenses, anxiety, and impulses with confrontation, clarification, and interpretation. It attempts to confront defensive behavior and elicit affect in an interpersonal context so that repressed memories and ideas are fully experienced, and both affect and ideas are consciously integrated. Brief adaptive therapy has somewhat of a more cognitive approach, focusing on identifying the patient's major maladaptive pattern and elucidating it in both past and present relationships, especially in the patient-therapist relationship. The aim is to enable the patient to develop insight into the origins and present determinants of the pattern, leading to better adapted interpersonal relationships. The authors documented that the intended differences in technique were in fact found (A. Winston et al. 1991). Both treatments produced overall equivalent results, but there were some differential results. Short-term dynamic psychotherapy produced better results in patients with an obsessional personality style, whereas brief adaptive therapy showed better results in those with a histrionic style (A. Winston et al. 1991). These results are consistent with the clinical observation that obsessional patients need help accessing affective experience and histrionic patients benefit from placing their experience in a cognitive framework.

Addressing Defenses

The patient's maladaptive defenses, or, more colloquially, defensiveness, may play a special role in responding to therapy. Foreman and Marmar (1985) described some patients who had initially poor alliances that improved, producing good outcomes when the therapists addressed their defenses and resistance. Gaston et al. (1988) found that higher degrees of defensiveness contributed to lower working alliance in behavioral, cognitive, and brief dynamic therapies for depression. In a study of the therapeutic process in their personality disorder sample, B. Winston et al. (1994) found that the therapist addressing defenses was highly correlated with change in target complaints.

Summary of Findings

Psychotherapy studies indicate that, as a group, personality disorders improve with treatment. This conclusion also has been reached in previous reviews (Perry et al. 1999; Reich and Vasile 1993; Roth and Fonagy 1996; Sanislow and McGlashan 1998; Shea 1993; Target 1998). On average, the effects of treatment are large—two to four times larger than improvement seen in control conditions. Limited randomized clinical treatment trials indicate that psychotherapy is significantly more efficacious than control conditions, such as a wait-list or treatment as usual in the community. This statement is strongest for self-reported but more suggestive for observer-rated improvement. Clearly, both the severity of the patient's disorder (Cluster B disorders are generally more severe than Cluster C disorders) and the other less well understood factors affect who improves and by how much. Although the degree of improvement is large on most measures, there is variation by a factor of two. Subjective complaints and volatile or state-dependent measures, such as depression or global functioning, register very large changes, whereas interpersonal and social role functioning, which are closer to core psychiatric disturbance, register lower degrees of improvement.

Remission or recovery from meeting full criteria for a personality disorder appears to be a function of the duration of treatment, in addition to the specific diagnosis or severity and other factors. Four studies suggested that a mean of 52% of patients, given one to two treatment sessions per week, experienced remission after about 1.3 years of treatment. Additional analysis in this review indicated that differences exist among personality types in their rates of recovery. Less is known about which patient and treatment factors are associated with remission or persistence of personality disorders. A model of the rate of change suggested that 25.8% of patients improved per year, but the model could not be extrapolated beyond about 70% remitted. This model contrasted with a previous model based on the naturalistic follow-up of borderline personality disorder, which found that 3.7% remitted per year. Both models might have had different results if the studies had included treatment dropouts with completers. Although these models should be considered hypotheses requiring further validation, they point to the need to consider longer- rather than shorter-term treatments for personality disorders.

Dropout from treatment varies from approximately 10% to 30% depending on treatment length. Less is known about which patients drop out because studies too often focus on only those completing treatment. However, patients with borderline personality disorder may be especially prone to drop out, as are those receiving group modalities as their sole therapy. One goal for developing treatments is the need to prevent dropout.

A good therapeutic alliance, or one that is improving, appears to characterize successful cases. The treatment recommendations and manuals of the future will likely focus the clinician's attention on the state of the alliance and how to address problems interfering with a better alliance. A good alliance is important for all personality disorders but may be absolutely crucial for more severe cases, especially borderline personality disorder and antisocial personality disorder, which one study suggested may be treatable only in the presence of a positive therapeutic alliance. Patients should be encouraged to continue a therapy long enough to address issues associated with a poor alliance, because even though we do not necessarily know what happens to dropouts, we do know that completers have a good chance at improvement. Nonetheless, there is no reason to endure a therapy characterized by a persistently poor alliance. In those instances, a change in therapist or therapy type may be in the patient's best interest.

The alliance is a product of the therapist-patient interaction; further research will help to elucidate its constituents. Patient factors include the severity of the personality disorder and basic aspects of personality, such as the level of defensive functioning and quality of object relations. Therapist factors include the adjustment of the interventions to the level of support or exploration, the degree of focal adherence versus more openness to other topics, and the focus on insight, affect, or addressing defenses. All of these areas are promising but require substantial further study. Thus, the manuals of the future will require a generation of research testing current clinical wisdom about how the therapist should adjust his or her therapeutic interventions based on the patient's functioning in a given session over the course of therapy.

Finally, despite the caveats about the limitations of the existing studies, our current level of knowledge is sufficient to warrant a message of hope: to patients seeking psychotherapy for personality disorders, that they can improve, and to their therapists, that empirical research may begin to lead rather than lag clinical wisdom and begin to offer directions on how better to help these patients.

References

Alden L: Short-term structured treatment for avoidant personality disorder. J Consult Clin Psychol 56:756–764, 1989

American Psychiatric Association: Diagnostic and Statistical Manual of Mental Disorders, 4th Edition. Washington, DC, American Psychiatric Association, 1994

Barber J: Change in obsessive-compulsive and avoidant personality disorders following dynamic psychotherapy. Psychotherapy 34:133–143, 1997

Bond M, Banon E, Grenier M: Differential effects of interventions on the therapeutic alliance with patients with personality disorders. J Psychother Pract Res 7:301–318, 1998

Budman S, Demby A, Soldz S, et al: Time-limited group psychotherapy for patients with personality disorders: outcomes and drop-outs. Int J Group Psychother 46:357–377, 1996

Diguer L, Barber J, Luborsky L: Three concomitants: personality disorders, psychiatric severity and outcome of dynamic psychotherapy of major depression. Am J Psychiatry 150:1246–1248, 1993

Dolan B, Warren F, Kingsley N: Change in borderline symptoms one year after therapeutic community treatment for severe personality disorder. Br J Psychiatry 171:274–279, 1997

Fahy TA, Eisler I, Russell GFM: Personality disorder and treatment response in bulimia nervosa. Br J Psychiatry 162:765–770, 1993

Foreman SA, Marmar CR: Therapist actions that address initially poor therapeutic alliances in psychotherapy. Am J Psychiatry 142:922–926, 1985

Gabbard GO (ed): Treatments of Psychiatric Disorders, 3rd Edition. Washington, DC, American Psychiatric Press (in press)

Gabbard GO, Horwitz L, Allen JG, et al: Transference interpretation in the psychotherapy of borderline patients: a high-risk, high-gain phenomenon. Harv Rev Psychiatry 2:59–69, 1994

Gaston L, Marmar CR, Thompson LW, et al: Relation of patient pretreatment characteristics to the therapeutic alliance in diverse psychotherapies. J Consult Clin Psychol 56:483–489, 1988

Gerstley L, McLellen AT, Alterman A, et al: Ability to form an alliance with a therapist: a possible marker of prognosis for patients with antisocial PD. Am J Psychiatry 146:508–512, 1989

Gunderson JG, Frank AF, Ronningstam EF, et al: Early discontinuance of borderline patients from psychotherapy. J Nerv Ment Dis 177:38–42, 1989

Hafner RJ, Holme G: The influence of a therapeutic community on psychiatric disorder. J Clin Psychol 52:461–468, 1996

Hardy GE, Barkham M, Shapiro DA, et al: Impact of cluster C personality disorders on outcomes of contrasting brief psychotherapies for depression. J Clin Consult Psychol 63:997–1004, 1995

Hilsenroth MJ, Holdwick DJ, Castlebury FD, et al: The effects of DSM-IV Cluster B personality disorder symptoms on the termination and continuation of psychotherapy. Psychotherapy 35:163–176, 1998

Hoglend P: Personality disorders and long-term outcome after brief dynamic psychotherapy. J Personal Disord 7:168–181, 1993

Hoglend P, Piper WE: Focal adherence in brief dynamic psychotherapy: a comparison of findings from two independent studies. Psychotherapy 32:618–628, 1995

Horvath AO, Luborsky L: The role of therapeutic alliance in psychotherapy. J Clin Consult Psychol 61:561–573, 1993

Karterud S, Vaglum S, Friis S, et al: Day hospital therapeutic community treatment for patients with personality disorders. J Nerv Ment Dis 180:238–243, 1992

Kernberg OF, Selzer M, Koenigsberg H: Psychodynamic Psychotherapy of Borderline Patients. New York, Basic Books, 1991, p 55

Kopta SM, Howard KI, Lowry JL, et al: Patterns of symptomatic recovery in psychotherapy. J Consult Clin Psychol 62:1009–1016, 1994

Krawitz R: A prospective psychotherapy outcome study. Aust N Z J Psychiatry 31:465–473, 1997

Krupnick J, Sotsky SM, Elkin I, et al: The role of the therapeutic alliance in psychotherapy and pharmacotherapy outcome: findings in the National Institute of Mental Health Treatment of Depression Collaborative Research Program. J Clin Consult Psychol 64:532–539, 1996

Liberman RP, Eckman T: Behavior therapy vs insight-oriented therapy for repeated suicide attempters. Arch Gen Psychiatry 38:1126–1130, 1981

Linehan MM: Cognitive-Behavioral Treatment of Borderline Personality Disorder. New York, Guilford, 1993, p 167

Linehan MM, Tutek BA, Heard HL, et al: Interpersonal outcome of cognitive behavioral treatment for chronically suicidal borderline patients. Am J Psychiatry 151:1771–1776, 1994

Marziali E, Munroe-Blum H, McCleary L: The contribution of group cohesion and group alliance to outcome of group psychotherapy. Int J Group Psychotherapy 47:475–497, 1997

Monsen JT, Odland T, Eilertsen DE: Personality disorders: changes and stability after intensive psychotherapy focusing on affect consciousness. Psychotherapy Research 5:33–48, 1995

Munroe-Blum H, Marziali E: A controlled trial of short-term group treatment for borderline personality disorder. J Personal Disord 9:190–198, 1995

Patience DA, McGuire RJ, Scott AI, et al: The Edinburgh Primary Care Study: personality disorder and outcome. Br J Psychiatry 167:324–330, 1995

Perry JC: Longitudinal studies of personality disorders. J Personal Disord 7 (suppl):63–85, 1993

Perry JC, Banon E, Ianni F: The effectiveness of psychotherapy for personality disorders. Am J Psychiatry 156:1312–1321, 1999

Piper WE, Azim HFA, Joyce AS, et al: Quality of object relations versus interpersonal functioning as predictors of therapeutic alliance and psychotherapy outcome. J Nerv Ment Dis 179:432–438, 1991

Piper WE, Rosie JS, Azim HFA, et al: A randomized trial of psychiatric day treatment for patients with affective and personality disorders. Hospital and Community Psychiatry 44:757–763, 1993

Piper WE, Boroto DR, Joyce AS, et al: Pattern of alliance and outcome in short-term individual psychotherapy. Psychotherapy 32:639–647, 1995

Reich JH, Vasile RG: Effect of personality disorders on the treatment of Axis I conditions: an update. J Nerv Ment Dis 181:475–484, 1993

Rosenthal RN, Muran JC, Pinsker H, et al: Interpersonal change in brief supportive psychotherapy. J Psychother Pract Res 8:55–63, 1999

Roth A, Fonagy P: What Works for Whom? A Critical Review of Psychotherapy Research. New York, Guilford, 1996, pp 197–215

Samsone RA, Fine MA, Dennis AB: Treatment impressions and termination experiences with borderline patients. Am J Psychotherapy 45:173–180, 1991

Sanislow CA, McGlashan TH: Treatment outcome of personality disorders. Can J Psychiatry 43:237–250, 1998

Shea MT: Psychosocial treatment of personality disorders. J Personal Disord 7 (suppl):167–180, 1993

Shea MT, Pilkonis PA, Beckham E, et al: Personality disorders and treatment outcome in the NIMH Treatment of Depression Collaborative Research Program. Am J Psychiatry 147:711–718, 1990

Skodol AE, Buckley P, Charles E: Is there a characteristic pattern to the treatment history of clinic outpatients with borderline personality? J Nerv Ment Dis 171:405–410, 1983

Stevenson J, Meares R: An outcome study of psychotherapy for patients with borderline personality disorder. Am J Psychiatry 149:358–362, 1992

Stone MH: Psychotherapy with schizotypal borderline patients. J Am Acad Psychoanal 11:87–111, 1983

Target M: Outcome research on the psychosocial treatment of personality disorders. Bull Menninger Clin 62:215–230, 1998

Vaillant GE, Perry JC: Personality disorders, in Comprehensive Textbook of Psychiatry, 3rd Edition. Edited by Kaplan HI, Freedman AH, Sadock BJ. Baltimore, MD, Williams & Wilkins, 1980, pp 1562–1590

Waldinger R, Gunderson JG: Completed psychotherapies with borderline patients. Am J Psychother 38:190–202, 1984

Wallerstein RS: The psychotherapy research project of the Menninger Foundation: an overview. J Clin Consult Psychol 57:195–205, 1989

Wilberg T, Karterud S, Urnes O, et al: Outcomes of poorly functioning patients with personality disorders in a day treatment program. Psychiatr Serv 49:1462–1467, 1998

Winston A, Pollack J, McCullough L, et al: Brief psychotherapy of personality disorders. J Nerv Ment Dis 179:188–193, 1991

Winston A, Laikin M, Pollack J, et al: Short-term psychotherapy of personality disorders. Am J Psychiatry 151:190–194, 1994

Winston B, Winston A, Samstag LW, et al: Patient defense/therapist interventions. Psychotherapy 31:478–491, 1994

Woody GE, McLellan T, Luborsky LL, et al: Sociopathy and psychotherapy outcome. Arch Gen Psychiatry 42:1081–1086, 1985

Yoemans FE, Gutfreund J, Selzer MA, et al: Factors related to drop-outs by borderline patients: treatment contract and therapeutic alliance. J Psychother Pract Res 3:16–24, 1994

Chapter 2

Psychodynamic Psychotherapy for Borderline Personality Disorder

John G. Gunderson, M.D.

The sheer magnitude of the literature on psychodynamic psychotherapies for borderline personality disorder precludes the possibility that this review can be other than selective. I deliberately omit subjects covered in other chapters in this volume, including the considerable research that has been done on outcome (see Perry and Bond, Chapter 1), the combination with pharmacotherapy (see Gabbard, Chapter 3), and the growing literature on cognitive therapies (see Tyrer and Davidson, Chapter 5). Primarily the clinical psychodynamic literature is reviewed here.

Defining Psychotherapy

Although the term *psychotherapy* can be used to encompass a broad range of psychosocial therapies, here it refers specifically to individual psychotherapies and, as noted, only those with a psychodynamic base. Beyond this, I believe it is necessary to distinguish psychotherapy from case management insofar as many of the problems in treating borderline personality disorder derive from misguided efforts to implement psychotherapies (i.e., assume a readiness with shared goals and collaborative intentions) for borderline patients who need more and other forms of treatment. Individual psychotherapies may begin while borderline patients are in a hospital, a residential setting, or an intensive outpatient program, but in the context of these levels of care, the role of individual psychotherapy often will be adjunctive, and the specific goals of psychotherapy (e.g., personal growth) will be secondary to the goals of case management (i.e., symptom relief and behavioral management).

The term *psychotherapy*, as used in this chapter, refers to a modality that is not primarily designed to stop "bad things" (i.e., to relieve symptoms or to diminish self-destructive or otherwise maladaptive behaviors). Although psychotherapy also can decrease symptoms or maladaptive behaviors, it is distinguished by its intention to do "good things" (i.e., to help patients change for the better—to develop new psychological capacities). As such, *treatments* differ from *therapies*. Treatments (e.g., medication, diet, hospitalization) are given to patients; a patient passively receives (or resists) but does not initiate them. Therapies require active participation, shared goals, and at least intermittent collaboration.

It is critical to the overall treatment program for borderline patients to have a primary clinician, someone who is responsible for safety and for overseeing the choice, implementation, coordination, and monitoring of the treatment components, but this role is not the same as that of a psychotherapist. This distinction is especially important for borderline patients because, in what is later identified as the first phase of treatment, most of them require significant amounts of management (noted as "treatment" in the previous paragraph) for manifest behavioral, mood, and cognitive problems. During the early phases of therapy, the primary clinician's administrative role has some inherent conflicts with the role of a dynamic psychotherapist (as is discussed later in this chapter in the section titled "Phase I: Building a Contractual Alliance").

Borderline patients often develop a readiness for psychotherapy out of working with someone who has had a case manager/primary clinician role. Indeed, someone who serves as a primary clinician may gradually move away from the case management role into a less administrative and more exploratory role, but it is increasingly common during the first phase for a psychotherapist's role to be separated (so-called split treatment). Split treatment can take many forms, but the most common one is when a psychopharmacologist rather than a psychotherapist also serves as the primary clinical case manager. Psychiatrists are apt to be involved in split treatments when they assume responsibilities for medication and case management activities, but the psychotherapist's role is often transferred to psychologists or members of other disciplines. The retreat from assuming the psychotherapeutic role by psychiatrists is, I believe, an unfortunate shift in services for borderline patients because the deeper knowledge of such patients that psychotherapeutic sessions allow can greatly inform pharmacotherapy and case management. Still, collaborative work among two or more treaters has definite advantages. When split treatments are collaborative, in my experience, they establish a better containment for splits and projections and thereby diminish dropouts (see Gunderson, in press).

Background

History

Psychoanalysts' initial descriptive accounts of borderline patients were largely prompted by the uniquely vexing clinical problems, such as testing boundaries and regressing in unstructured settings, that characteristically occurred in psychoanalytic therapies. When Kernberg (1968) and Masterson (1971, 1972) wrote surprisingly optimistic reports about the treatability of these patients, they inspired a tide of long-term psychoanalytically informed inpatient and outpatient treatments. Since 1968, 53 books have been written about psychoanalytic psychotherapies with borderline patients (Library of Congress database search). These psychotherapies usually have been initiated with ambitious hopes for curative or at least basic structural changes in the disordered personality.

Well before the swell of enthusiasm for intensive long-term psychoanalytic psychotherapies was cresting in the early 1980s, the excesses, limitations, and narrowness of this approach were being recorded. Many clinicians, including notable analysts (Freidman 1975; Zetzel 1971), believed that intensive or long-term psychotherapeutic interventions were often unnecessarily regressive. In the 1980s, Waldinger and Gunderson (1984, 1989) had shown that dramatic success, although possible, was rare. Throughout this period, the ongoing debates within the psychoanalytic psychotherapy community helped winnow out bad ideas and helped to more firmly establish the areas of concordance.

The reservations about psychoanalytic therapies were reinforced by changing tides within psychiatry and the health care system during the 1980s and 1990s. Psychiatry's move to paradigms that were both more biological and more scientific encouraged skepticism about psychoanalytically based therapies that were psychological and without empirical support. Biological psychiatrists presented real antagonism to psychoanalytic claims, and the scientific reforms led to treatments that were increasingly disorder-specific and empirically validated. Psychiatric training increasingly narrowed the role of psychotherapists into a career track to be selected rather than the major modality in which competence would determine credentialing. So the treatment of borderline patients became multifaceted, increasingly requiring a team approach and increasingly moving psychotherapy into an elective strategy rather than a sine qua non of treatment.

At present, psychotherapy is central to long-term treatment plans, but its role is qualified: it takes its place alongside other modalities, it is better for some borderline patients than for others, and it should be practiced only by those with special qualifications.

Utilization

Without question, individual psychotherapies have been the cornerstone of treatment for borderline personality disorder. In a recent study of 158 borderline patients selected from multiple clinical sites, more than 90% had received individual psychotherapy, and the mean length of their prior psychotherapy was 51 months (Bender et al., submitted), although some of what these patients call "psychotherapy" doubtlessly includes what might more accurately be referred to as administrative or case management functions. This finding is all the more remarkable for having occurred within a managed-care environment in which such lengths of treatment are actively discouraged. In other research, outpatients with borderline personality disorder reported a mean of six prior psychotherapists (Perry et al. 1990; Skodol et al. 1983).

Having noted these findings, it is nonetheless my impression that the modern mental health care system's movement toward empirically supported treatments and eclecticism is systematically reducing the frequency with which long-term psychodynamic psychotherapies are being initiated.

Patient and Therapist "Readiness" for Psychotherapy

Patient Characteristics

In 1982, Kernberg wrote a review of psychodynamic therapies. In an effort to distinguish patients who were suitable (i.e., for whom psychodynamic psychotherapies were indicated), he noted motivation, psychological mindedness, and capacity for introspection. Table 2–1 revisits this in terms of "readiness," citing seeing problems in oneself and wanting to change. Kernberg also warned against patients with significant antisocial problems or too much reliance on secondary gain (again, motivational issues) or those who have such extreme situational instability or impulsivity that these issues would preoccupy their treatment. These issues are framed in Table 2–1 as needing to be able to take adequate responsibility for their own safety. To be clear, this does not mean that borderline patients who willfully endanger themselves are not good candidates for dynamic therapy; it excludes only those whose safety issues are so frequent, dangerous, and impulsive that their meaning would not be accessible.

Table 2–1. Readiness for psychotherapy

Patient	Therapist
Sees problem in self	Trained in skills that facilitate change
Seeks change that is desirable	Agrees with patient's goals for change
Patient (or others) in principle can assume primary responsibility for patient's safety	Can contain patient's/own emotions but does not ensure patient's safety

Therapist Characteristics

To my knowledge, no research has helped to characterize desirable qualities in psychodynamic psychotherapists for borderline patients. Certainly, in my experience, therapists' aptitudes vary considerably. Pfohl (1999) recently showed that some psychiatrists, many social workers, and most nurses recognize that they are not "good for borderline patients" and would happily avoid them. Yet many mental health professionals do not recognize this or believe that they are capable but are not in fact "good for borderline patients." Being blind to one's limitations may be based on naiveté (about oneself or about borderline patients), but it is also pushed by the appeal (Main 1957) such patients can have for prospective therapists (i.e., the promise of being very helpful to someone for whom life has been unfair and whom others have failed). But being blind to one's limitations also can be propelled by the very practical pressures to fill one's time—whether in private practice or in a clinic. Pfohl's study (1999) indicated that as a discipline, psychologists proved distinctly—and quite uniformly—more optimistic about the borderline patient's likely responsiveness to psychotherapies. Mental health professionals who had more administrative experience in hospital or residential programs had less polarized ideas.

To become "good with borderline patients" as a psychotherapist requires experience, training, and, I believe, certain personal qualities. With respect to experience, developing comfort and competence with borderline patients usually requires 2–3 years of fairly extensive, preferably multifaceted, contacts such as those derived from work within inpatient and residential settings. Psychiatrists who manage medications for many borderline outpatients also can learn such basic comfort and competence. Such experiences make one comfortable with the management issues typifying early phases of treatment.

If an otherwise good therapist wants to learn the special psychotherapeutic skills required to become "good with borderline patients," the training requires good supervision for several cases over the course of the first 1–2 years of treatment (when management issues are prominent). Only psychiatrists or psychologists

Table 2–2. Therapist's attitudes necessary to take on a borderline patient

- Believes the patient is interested (e.g., challenging, touching, confusing, attractive, needy, smart)
- Believes the patient can improve
- Accepts that he or she may be essential for the patient's welfare— a serious responsibility
- Perceives the patient sympathetically (hostilities, acting out, and symptoms occur for a reason)
- Believes that he or she can help
- Is prepared to persevere despite needing to do things he or she does not want to do or being criticized or hurt
- Is ready to work with others and to use supervision or consultation

who have already seen borderline patients nonintensively with good psychodynamic supervision and who then undertake advanced psychotherapeutic training are good candidates to do intensive psychoanalytic therapies with properly selected borderline patients—*if* they have good supervision.

Beyond experience and training, becoming "good with borderline patients" involves a therapist's personal qualities of character and attitude (i.e., what has been disparagingly considered a nonspecific component of what therapists offer). It is not merely a matching issue. Therapists who do well with one borderline patient will do well with most. Therapists who do not find the issues that surround the treatment of borderline patients interesting (i.e., action, dependency, anger) or who do not actually like such patients will be unlikely to do well with them. They are unlikely to find that exceptional borderline patient with whom they will be able to work well. Table 2–2 identifies attitudes I believe increase the likelihood of a therapist doing well with borderline patients.

In addition to these attitudes, some characterological traits are important for success. Therapists who do well are usually reliable, somewhat adventurous, action-oriented, and good-humored. This translates into being active and responsive. Therapists who are unlikely to do well are effete, genteel, passive, or controlling. Kernberg and Linehan may exemplify personal qualities of therapists who are good with borderline patients. Both are authoritative, confident, forceful, and clear. Swenson (1989) noted that both Linehan and Kernberg meet "the patient's emotional intensity and lability head-on with steady emotional intensity of her own. Both therapists give the patient the feeling that they are present, engaged, and indestructible. The patient feels emotionally held" (p. 32). My guess is that patients feel moved to accept what these therapists say to them for the same reasons that many professionals want to do as they suggest. Moreover, both Kernberg and Linehan seem undaunted by controversy but challenged certainly, perhaps even enjoying debate and disagreement. No doubt borderline patients are impressed by their readiness to offer their viewpoints, by their efforts to make themselves clear, and by their attention to fine distinctions. I suspect that patients find that both listen carefully and seem clearly engaged by them. Patients of either Kernberg or Linehan will, I believe, feel confident that their opinions, judgments, or decisions will be heard and responded to, what Swenson summarized as feeling "emotionally held" (p. 32). I believe that these personal qualities are often found in therapists who are in fact good with borderline patients.

Phases of Therapy

Overview

Alliance Building

The concept of a therapeutic alliance helps to frame the discussion of both initiation of individual psychotherapy in borderline patients and the longer-term processes within such therapies. The concept has special significance for borderline personality disorder insofar as at one time it was considered a necessary prerequisite for therapy that rendered many such patients unsuitable (see Adler 1979). To guide our use of the term, Table 2–3 adopts definitions of three types that have appeared to occur sequentially during therapy (Greenspan and Scharfstein 1981; Luborsky 1976).

Table 2–3. Three forms of therapeutic alliance

1. **Contractual (behavioral):** initial agreement between the patient and therapist on treatment goals and their roles in achieving them (phase I)

2. **Relational (affective/empathic):** emphasized by Rogerian client-centered relationships; patient experiences the therapist as caring, understanding, genuine, and likable (phase II)

3. **Working (cognitive/motivational):** psychoanalytic prototype; patient joins the therapist as a reliable collaborator to help the patient understand herself or himself; its development represents a significant improvement for borderline patients (phases III–IV)

To a considerable extent, the problems of dropouts can be diminished by giving special attention to mutually agreed on expectations for the therapy. This is done by defining roles and goals and by establishing a concrete framework. This process forms the earliest form of alliance, the *contractual* alliance.

Several studies have examined the alliance between borderline patients and their therapists. In the McLean prospective repeated-measures study of 35 patients with borderline personality disorder who were beginning individual psychotherapies, the alliance improved steadily over a period of years (Gunderson et al. 1997). In the Menninger Treatment Intervention Project, the long-term course of the alliance did not show similar overall improvement, but audiotapes revealed that the level of alliance within sessions fluctuated dramatically throughout the therapies (Gabbard et al. 1988, 1994; Horwitz et al. 1996). Of note, in both studies the initial alliance scores were higher than expected.

Generic Sequence of Change

To develop treatment goals and to assess whether existing treatments are making timely progress, an overall conceptual framework for processes of change is essential. Emerging from my own experience and supported by a review of related literature (Kopta et al. 1994; Lanktree and Briere 1995) is a fairly predictable sequence in which changes can be expected. As noted by Perry and Bond (see Chapter 1 in this volume), findings from

Table 2–4. Framework for expected changes

Areas of disturbance	Relevant interventions	Expected time for change
Subjective state	Concerned attention, validation, interpretation	Weeks
Dysphoric feelings	Reality testing	
	Problem solving	
	Pattern recognition	
Behavior	Clarification of defensive purpose and maladaptive consequences	Months
Interpersonal style	Confrontation	6–18 months
	Pattern recognition	
	Here-and-now interactional analysis	
Intrapsychic organization	Defense and transference analysis	>2 years
	Corrective relationships, real relationships	

Source. Reprinted from Gunderson JG, Gabbard GO: "Making the Case for Psychoanalytic Therapies in the Current Psychiatric Environment." *J Am Psychoanal Assoc* 47:695, 1999. Used with permission.

research with personality disorder patients also support the framework for the expected changes seen in Table 2–4. The examination of five successfully treated borderline patients (Gunderson et al. 1993; Waldinger and Gunderson 1989) showed a sequence of changes and a timetable that are consistent with this framework. In the first few years of treatment, family interventions can successfully reduce family tensions (Berkowitz et al., in press), and partial hospital services can reduce self-destructiveness and depression within the first year (Bateman and Fonagy 1999). First-stage targets for dialectical behavior therapy are grossly maladaptive behaviors (Linehan 1993). Next are stress tolerance and self-care and then third-stage targets that involve intrapsychic objectives such as increased self-respect and pursuit of individual goals.

Phases of Change

Table 2–5 offers a sequence and approximate timetable for changes within successful intensive (two or more sessions per week) psychotherapies with borderline patients. This table reflects a revision and refinement of my previous efforts (i.e., Gunderson 1984; Gunderson et al. 1997; Waldinger and Gunderson 1989). In some ways, it mirrors the generic stages of change already described but elaborates on how these changes apply to borderline patients and how they are facilitated by processes within psychotherapy. The timeline may vary considerably (e.g., for patients with poor social aptitude or significant secondary gain, it may take 2 years to move into phase III), but the sequence by which changes occur is quite predictable. It is important to recognize that there are significant variations in terms of which stage borderline patients start from (e.g., some are very unaware of anger and some are successfully employed).

The clinical value of tentatively proposing such a sequence and timetable of expectable changes is that therapists, patients, or families can then more comfortably recognize that failure to see such changes raises questions about effectiveness. This does not mean that such therapies are not beneficial. It means that the question should be raised whether the therapeutic services could be improved. The best way to address these issues is by consultation. In summary, Table 2–5 offers a "big picture" scheme; individual borderline patients vary, and all will shift back and forth in their functioning. The table is used as a guide for the following description of the phases of change.

Phase I: Building a Contractual Alliance (see Table 2–5)

Dropouts

A series of studies initiated in the 1980s documented very high dropout rates (43%–67%) of borderline patients from psychotherapies. In a study of 60 borderline patients who were beginning psychotherapies at McLean Hospital in Belmont, Massachusetts, the most common reasons for dropping out were 1) too much frus-

Table 2–5. Indices of change in long-term psychotherapies

	Phase I (0–3 months)	Phase II (1 month–1 year)	Phase III (1–2 or 3 years)	Phase IV (2 or 3 years–?)	Result
Change target	→ Symptoms (moods)	→ Self-destructiveness → Impulsivity	→ Maladaptive interpersonal problems → Projection	→ Splitting → owning anger → Avoidance	→ Emptiness ← Friends
Therapeutic relationship	Contractual alliance: • agreed-on goals and roles • counterdependent	Relational alliance: • therapist valued • dependent/anxious	Relational alliance: • *therapy* valued • dependent/positive	Working alliance: • separation anxiety	Secure attachment
Major issues	Action, symptoms, fearfulness Anger and denial of anger Projection	Affect recognition and tolerance Accepting neediness Anger projected	Misattribution, assertiveness Fear of aggression Anger projected	Negative transference Re-entering competition Developmental issues: trauma, self-image	Internal locus of control

Table 2–5. Indices of change in long-term psychotherapies *(continued)*

	Phase I (0–3 months)	Phase II (1 month–1 year)	Phase III (1–2 or 3 years)	Phase IV (2 or 3 years–?)	Result
Therapist activities	Interactive, responsive, educates and clarifies	Clarifies maladaptive responses to feelings (e.g., frustration); validates and empathizes; develops formulation	Identifies conflicts and misattributions; supports functional capabilities; connects present to past	Interprets conflicts and transference; confronts avoidance	Not applicable
Outcome	Patient likes and is engaged by therapist	Capable of low-demand social role	Capable of low-demand relationships	Capable of competition, friendships	Not borderline personality disorder

Source. Reprinted from Gunderson JG: *Treatment of Borderline Personality Disorder.* Washington, DC, American Psychiatric Press (in press). Used with permission.

tration, 2) lack of family support, and 3) logistics (travel, time, costs) (Gunderson et al. 1989). Notably, neither the patients nor the therapists in this study were preselected for suitability for psychotherapy. In another study that surveyed senior and expert therapists, we found a similar pattern (Waldinger and Gunderson 1984). This survey indicated that even the experts have problems keeping borderline patients engaged in psychotherapy—of 790 borderline patients, 54% continued psychotherapy beyond 6 months, and only 33% went on to complete their therapy satisfactorily. These studies have made it clear that engaging borderline patients in individual psychotherapy is difficult, and whatever role individual psychotherapy might hold, it will often be unfulfilled insofar as about half will leave before its benefits could be expected.

Psychotherapy Contracts

As described earlier in this chapter, the contractual alliance (see Table 2–3) is an agreement between the patient and the clinician about goals and their respective roles. This agreement includes practical issues such as fees, payment scheduling, attendance, and confidentiality. While creating this alliance, the therapist establishes a frame for the therapy that represents the therapist's professionalism and boundaries. The "frames" of the therapy are the obvious signs that the therapist is a professional at work—work that involves discipline, expectations, and restraints.

In an effort to engage borderline patients in psychotherapy more successfully, Kernberg's group formalized the process of creating a contract (Selzer et al. 1987). Akhtar (1982), like Kernberg et al. (1989), used contracting to create an agreed-on frame that can be referred to when problems are encountered so that the frame does not then seem arbitrary, reactive, or punitive. Linehan (1993) also places great significance on establishing a contract for borderline patients before starting dialectical behavior therapy (e.g., establishing clear goals for change and making a commitment to attend regularly).

These clinicians may use multiple sessions, almost always at least two, to reach an agreement about the roles and goals before therapy is begun. Spending time on developing such a contract is consistent with one of the overall considerations about the role of individual psychotherapies for borderline patients. Dynamic psychotherapies that rely heavily on a patient's ability to control impulses and that invite affect expression often require strengths that are unusual in many borderline patients, strengths that may need to have been attained by other concurrent or preceding types of therapy. Indeed, in the absence of such strengths, other therapies, including dialectical behavior therapy, medication, and case management, may need to take precedence.

Yeomans et al. (1992) emphasized that the contract should be explicit about the limits of the therapist's role and responsibilities; for example, "it does not fall within the role of the therapist to get involved in the action of a patient's life through phone calls, emergency room visits, etc." (p. 256). This delimitation of the therapist's role (reflecting the viewpoint of Kernberg et al. 1989) stems from a conviction that a therapist's involvement with the patient's life outside of sessions is frequently the cause of treatment failures. Yeomans et al. (1992, 1993) noted that the contract begins with a statement by the therapist about the minimal conditions under which therapy can be conducted and that this statement is followed by a dialogue that invites the patient to respond. During the dialogue, again at the therapist's initiative, problems are anticipated based on the patient's history (e.g., coming to sessions intoxicated, having intersession crises, or not wanting to leave the session).

Although I find the idea of a contract generally helpful, it has some significant drawbacks. The most important is that many borderline patients are neither reliable nor foresighted enough to broker a meaningful contract. It also can introduce what may be an unnecessarily defensive and adversarial tone to the therapy.

I prefer to limit "contracting" to an agreement about practical issues, usually behavioral or interpersonal, and a few simple statements about the therapist's role. For example, I often say, "I see my role as helping you to understand yourself. I believe that will allow you to change." I then would cite some issues that arose during our evaluation sessions that seemed to have troubled the patient and that I foresee as amenable to change. I underscore, as does Linehan, that change is expected—that change is the explicit measure by which I judge, and encourage patients to judge,

Table 2–6. Relation between frequency of visits and goals

Frequency/week	Goals
1	Management grows into support; this can be an "anchor" (i.e., a stabilizing influence) that helps the patient to learn and grow from life experiences.
2	Sufficient for management and "therapy"—can foster change via insight by using either dynamic or cognitive strategies.
3	Optimal for dynamic therapies when examination of relationship is central. Personal growth can occur by virtue of therapy.
≥4	The patient's life is likely to revolve around therapy until growth; can be useful for patients who need an object but has significant potential for being harmful.

whether therapy is a worthwhile investment of our time and their money. I specifically would not tell a prospective or new borderline patient that I am not available except for emergencies or explain how he or she can expect me to respond to boundary issues. If a patient's behavior potentially endangers therapy (e.g., missing appointments, yelling) or safety (e.g., cutting, misusing medications), it should of course be addressed (but would not otherwise be taken up by the therapist), and it should be addressed without setting anticipatory limits.

Frequency and Goals

Table 2–6 indicates the relation between frequency of visits and therapeutic goals. Two or more psychotherapy sessions per week probably are required to correct unstable introjects or a pattern of insecure attachments, although this is untested. Kernberg et al. (1989) also advocate a minimum of twice-weekly appointments for psychodynamic therapies to be capable of effecting structural change (although they emphasize the requirements for transference analysis more than the requirements for the relationship per se to have corrective potential). Therapies with the mandate to help patients understand themselves, on which psychodynamic therapies rest, almost always require more than once-weekly sessions. The exception to this general rule is that the goals of dynamic therapy are feasible in once-weekly sessions when the therapist sees a patient who is being "held" by attending residential or intensive outpatient services three or more times per week.

If, however, the patient is seen once per week *in the absence of other modalities,* the therapist must provide the "holding" functions (i.e., become involved in crisis management, emergency telephone calls, medications, and other "reality" issues in which the therapist's involvement has great transference meaning but will go inadequately understood). The therapist's activities will require enough directives, advice, limits, and so on that the task is better labeled as "case management," and the role is what I have identified as that of the primary clinician. It is misleading to call this "psychotherapy," and the clinician might consider either reduced frequency or reduced duration of sessions.

Phase II: Building a Relational Alliance (see Table 2–5)

After a contractual alliance has been established and the patient has been engaged in therapy, a second phase of therapy begins in which the primary learning process involves mood and behavioral control and the development of a relational alliance (see Table 2–3). The relational alliance involves establishing a therapist's likability, dependability, and the perception that there is hope for a better future.

The Menninger Psychotherapy Research Project offers empirical data that help identify key therapeutic processes. This study distinguished between two types of psychotherapy: *expressive* (investigative, insight-oriented, emotion-generating) and *supportive* (directive, defense-reinforcing, emotion-inhibiting). Kernberg and colleagues' (1972) original interpretation, buttressed by Guttman's formidable statistical techniques, was that the data indicated that expressive techniques were effective. A reanalysis by Horwitz (1974) suggested that patients with borderline personality organization who received supportive therapy and who had a strong therapeutic alliance improved significantly. Wallerstein's (1986) further reanalysis of the data indicated that in actual practice, almost all the therapies offered a less expressive (i.e., less psychoanalytic) and more supportive approach than the study design had called for. Moreover, patients frequently switched between treatment modes and between therapists. Whereas Kernberg has persisted in viewing expressive insight-based therapy as superior, for Wallerstein and others, the results of this study have pointed toward the critical role of the supportive relational elements in treating borderline personality disorder.

Data supporting Wallerstein's interpretation come from two other sources. The Menninger Treatment Intervention Project found that although patients' receptivity to expressive techniques varies over time, supportive elements are needed (Gabbard et al. 1994; Horwitz et al. 1996). Of further note is the significance of relational factors emphasized in the dramatically effective 1-year psychodynamic therapy studied by Stevenson and Meares (1992). Their brand of therapy was born of the Kohutian/Adlerian self psychological school, which emphasized empathic connection. The exploratory component of the therapy focused on the identification of the inevitable triggers that could disrupt the patient's sense of connectedness. These empirical sources of evidence reinforce Wallerstein's and Adler's conclusions (and my own clinical impressions) that supportive, attachment-generating interventions (as opposed to interpretative or confrontative intervention) are critically important in the early phases of successful psychotherapies. Notably, Linehan (1997; Linehan et al. 1991) gave comparatively modest reference to the therapeutic power of relational factors, but she did identify empathy and validation as critical components of dialectical behavior therapy.

The evidence thus becomes increasingly compelling that supportive empathic interventions are critically important in the second phase of psychotherapy. In the following section, I describe three components—identification of feelings, validation, and insight into interpersonal needs—that may facilitate the development of a relational alliance and prepare a patient for the later phases of change.

Identification of Feelings

The primary therapeutic techniques that make a relational alliance possible involve showing interest, conveying feasible expectations, showing resilience in the face of opposition, and, above all, as emphasized by Adler (1985) and demonstrated by Stevenson and Meares (1992), deploying empathy and validation. Empathy involves identification of a patient's dilemmas (e.g., "what a difficult situation" or "I can see why you were undecided") and especially of their feeling states (e.g., "you must have been scared" or "you seem angry about that"). This identification is often complicated by a patient's fears that such feelings are evidence of their "badness" or will be unacceptable to others. Fonagy and Target (1996) emphasized the corrective power of such interventions for those borderline patients whose feelings as children were ignored, mislabeled, or renounced. They learn to observe themselves by being observed—to paraphrase Winnicott, they "discover themselves in their mother's [or therapist's] eyes." They also learn a useful new way to label and accept part of their experience.

Although borderline patients' initial reaction to feedback about themselves is likely to be ambivalent, usually suspicious, and sometimes hostile, it helps to start by making observations at the surface. Uninvited observations indicate that the therapist is attending to the task of helping them learn about themselves. I often comment about facial expressions: "you look worried" or "you seemed sad when you talked about…" Actively identifying a patient's apparent feeling is most important when the patient looks either fearful or angry; both of these feelings may be difficult to recognize or talk about, and if overlooked, either can result in flight. Affirmation or disclosure by therapists about their own feelings, done with discretion, also assists this process of "mentalizing." For example, I almost always tell borderline patients about my feelings after any incident involving their safety issues. "It horrifies me to hear you describe cutting" or "I feel helpless" or "I felt really 'jerked around' after I got off the phone with your badly frightened boyfriend." Such disclosures help patients to represent feelings in their minds and the nonbehavioral ways they can affect others. It also presages a very important, recurring thematic process in long-term therapies whereby borderline patients connect behavior to events, to feelings, and to their thoughts.

Validation

Validation involves actively reinforcing the reality of borderline patients' perceptions and identifying the adaptive functions served by their defenses and behaviors. Of particular delicacy is the balance between listening sympathetically to disclosures of past mistreatment and, while validating the experience of unfairness, not assuming the validity of the realities as described (Gunderson and Chu 1993). It can be difficult not to offer validation for past mistreatment because the borderline patient often clearly wants that and because of the natural impulse to sympathize after such accounts. It is usually sufficient to convey that their life sounds like it was awful and that you can understand why under such circumstances they behave the way they characteristically do.

Insight Into Interpersonal Needs

Valuing a therapist usually results from a therapist's empathy and validation. These activities make a "good object" of the therapist. In contrast, valuing *therapy* derives from learning experiences. Interpretations or confrontations that bring to the patient's attention problems in himself or herself risk the therapist's becoming a "bad object." Still, by 3 or 6 months, the value of the tasks in therapy should be evident in the patients' reports that they have learned new things about themselves (Gunderson et al. 1997). Indeed, I like to underscore the therapy's task (i.e., understanding oneself) from the very first session by making observations about a patient and inquiring about whether he or she has learned anything new.

The central issue in the development of insight during phase II involves helping borderline patients understand how their wishes for caring attention prompt the interpersonal demands and evoke the rejections or anger that they fear. Nowhere is this issue more important than with the therapist (i.e., helping patients accept that their wish for caring attention is understandable and acceptable and that having those wishes be frustrated prompts many of their behavioral problems). Although this sounds like transference analysis, it is usually first identified in situations outside the therapy (e.g., "I knew when your mother went on vacation that you were likely to start drinking" or "when you leave the halfway house, as much as you hate it, it is going to represent a big loss for you"). Such interpretations about a patient's wish for nurturing attention underscore the therapist's role as an interested observer. When interpretations are met with hostility, the patient's feelings must be respected, but a therapist should not be apologetic (i.e., making observations is essential to a therapist's ability to be helpful). Indeed, I offer such observations in a psychoeducational way and support my observations by citing that such patterns of response are well known and familiar. In this way, the "interpretation" is neutralized, much in the way I believe Benjamin (1993) would combine education with dynamic formulation.

Obviously, the belief held by many borderline patients that "psychotherapy might help" after 6 months is enhanced by advances made in the relational alliance and by any actual learning that has taken place. Although the former is essential, it should never be considered sufficient. Continued involvement and investment by the therapist—as demonstrated by reliability, interest, and good judgment—evoke hope about the relationship that in the first phase of treatment is often experienced as dangerous vulnerability (e.g., "I'll get hurt, rejected,..."). Still, most borderline patients consciously entertain the idea some, if not most, of the time that "this therapist cares." By the end of the year, the patient should be involved in therapy and attached to the therapist (Table 2–5). This is another sign that the patient has achieved the goals of the second phase.

Phase III: Positive Dependency (see Table 2–5)

Between 6 and 18 months of therapy, as has been shown in the previous examinations of successful therapies (Waldinger and Gunderson 1989; Wallerstein 1986), positive dependency should have evolved. "Dependency" usually does not mean wanting to be told what to do; it primarily involves extreme sensitivity to the therapist's moods, attitudes, and absences. The patient here typically confesses that "my therapist means too much," thereby reflecting dependency and apprehension about it. This type of relationship also can be established with nondynamic and nonintensive clinicians, such as cognitive-behavioral therapists, case managers, or psychopharmacologists, but in these relationships, the dependency is more apt to involve actual direction and reassurance.

Under these circumstances, patients are less resistant to self-disclosure and more responsive to learning from a therapist's observations. Many of the testing behaviors and boundary problems that characterized the first year are significantly diminished. The work of connecting feelings to situations and behaviors remains central. Similarly, the theme of having needs for caring attention, and how frustration of those needs can be managed without action, recurs. These issues now can be addressed more easily within the context of the patient's responses to the therapist. In this period in the therapy, the exchanges can be quite intense, and a therapist's composure and containment usually can provide the needed holding without needing to step out of the therapist's role into case management activities ("parameters") or without needing to introduce a second modality. Learning to think about the relation of cause and effect, with respect to both feelings and interpersonal relationships, introduces delays over impulse discharge or avoidance. It helps build affect tolerance. Being able to conceptualize—the process that Fonagy terms *mentalization*—like any new habit, requires much repetition to become internalized (psychologically) or imbedded as new neural circuits (biologically) (Fonagy and Target 1996).

The Menninger study of alliance included a microanalysis of taped sessions for 39 patients with borderline personality disorder that documented multiple shifts in the level of collaboration (working alliance) within sessions (Allen et al. 1990). This work showed that advances apparent at one point in a session or even over longer periods will be dramatically reversed and then slowly regained. Nevertheless, I believe that the ontogeny of the therapy alliance is a dialectic process in which the more mature working forms progressively become more resilient and persistent while the regressions become less long-lived and less dramatic. Within this interactive process, broad generalizations can be made about the time frame by which signs of a developing alliance should be noted. In phase II, this involves the ability to hear feedback without flight and to "think about it." The absence of such signs once phase I ends is sufficiently troublesome that the viability and effectiveness of the therapy becomes questionable. For therapists, as Gabbard et al. (1994) pointed out, the rapidly alternating attitudes within sessions require therapists to be similarly deft, resourceful, and adaptive in their responses. In particular, they noted that interpretations are "high-risk, high-gain" interventions. This is especially true for the transference interpretations believed by Kernberg to be central.

An ongoing active review of what transpires in sessions in the interaction between patient and therapist is of significant value in helping patients gain cognitive and verbal means of processing the hurts and confusion caused by projections, misunderstandings, and intense feelings. The consistent review within sessions of what was said, meant, and so forth can be usefully supplemented by tape-recording sessions, a technique introduced by Martin Orne to help Sylvia Plath (who probably had borderline personality disorder). Tape-recording is sometimes resisted, but once begun, borderline patients usually are quite responsive to what they can learn. In addition to the specific clarification of "what really occurred" that recordings allow (it is very nice to have a borderline patient volunteer that she or he understood what you said or why you said it), the tapes serve as concrete extensions of the therapist's involvement and attention between sessions (i.e., as transitional objects; Winnicott 1953).

Therapists should expect that they will be transitional objects and then try to make the "silent" functions that they serve as explicit as possible. Thus, for example, just as the therapist's talk in the first year was helping the patient to understand that his or her actions stemmed from feelings and relational needs, in this second year, it will be valuable for the therapist to help the patient to identify what the patient "depends" on the therapist for. The essential component of this process involves issues of not being alone and of feeling connected—in effect, issues involving object constancy. Being able to recognize this will make it more easily managed. Table 2–7 indicates a hierarchy of ways to manage prolonged separations from therapists. Although interpretation of intolerance of aloneness runs the risk of imposing theory on a patient's experience, it is worth doing early and often because awareness of this dilemma can so effectively diminish unneces-

Table 2–7. Hierarchy of transitional options for use during therapist absences[a]

1. **Therapist accessible by telephone**
   Call as needed
   Call prescheduled

2. **Therapist substitutes: coverage by colleagues**
   Prescheduled meetings
   Meetings to be requested by the patient as needed

3. **Therapist-associated transitional objects**
   Tape-recorded sessions
   Notes from the therapist
   Cognitive-behavioral directives ("what to do")
   Items from the therapist's office

4. **Self-initiated coverage options**
   Increased contact with friends or relatives
   Increased social networking (e.g., events, clubs)
   Distracting oneself (e.g., travel, movies)

[a]These options are generally needed only for absences of more than a week. Options are listed hierarchically from most soothing to least soothing.
Source. From Gunderson JG: "The Borderline Patient's Intolerance of Aloneness: Insecure Attachments and Therapist Availability." *Am J Psychiatry* 153:757, 1996. Copyright 1996, the American Psychiatric Association. Reprinted by permission.

sary regressive responses and unnecessarily heroic acts of availability by therapists (see Gunderson 1996).

Still, most interpretive or confrontative activity in phase III remains in the domain of connecting feelings and behaviors to interpersonal situations. Even though this activity occurs increasingly within the relationship with the therapist, it does not quite conform to transference interpretations—it is learning to know oneself in new ways, not "about" oneself or why. The conclusion of phase III can occur as early as 2 years and usually occurs by year 3. At this point, the borderline patient has acquired a capacity for stable supportive relationships and for stable low-demand work (see Table 2–5). The borderline patient will remain insecure about rejections, fearful about separations, and prone to cut, drink, binge, rage, or withdraw in the face of conflicts. Such reactions are less severe and less prolonged than before therapy or during phase I. Patients will still be unable to rely on a consistent inner locus of control and will remain too reactive (defiant or compliant) with external pressures.

Phase IV: Becoming Nonborderline (see Table 2–5)

In phase IV, the psychotherapeutic techniques are no longer very specific to the borderline patient's psychopathology, except that the issues remain those unique to this diagnostic group. This phase is the least essential for mental rehabilitation, and it is of the most indefinite duration (see Table 2–5).

A stable and increasingly secure relationship has formed, and a collaborative working alliance generally can be assumed. The capacity for a secure attachment to the therapist may at last become evident, meaning an attachment in which absences may cause anxiety or objection but do not require substitutes or any therapist-associated objects (see Table 2–7). The relationship is no longer contaminated by fears of rejection or abandonment, and criticisms, although unwanted, can be responded to effectively.

The direct expression of hatefulness at the therapist that in Kernberg's theory is needed to remedy core psychopathology may occur during this phase. This remains, in my experience, a critical process in rendering a borderline patient nonborderline. This process is not always possible: deeply ingrained moralistic prohibitions, deficient intellectual/organizational capabilities, or fears about a therapist's destructibility (vulnerability) all can prevent this. Nor does this process usually occur in the cathartic way that I had imagined. Rather, it is more likely to occur in the form of direct and sometimes cruel indictments over long periods for which the therapist has become a safe container.

In this phase of therapy, long-denied problems with early trauma can be revisited usefully, or the developmental regions of distortions in body image can be explored. Such issues may take years to open up and to gain the needed desensitization or resolution. This process involves a patient's obtaining a coherent narrative of his or her life without major gaps, thereby consolidating a sense of self.

Entering competition is always desirable and conflictual for borderline patients because it triggers fears of aggression and of rejection. In addition to clarifying such fears, therapists often need to actively urge borderline patients to compete. Competition requires that borderline patients take initiatives on their own behalf without guilt; being autonomous and not apologetic are hard-won achievements for someone who has been borderline. The acquisition of stable, nonsexual, intimate relationships is almost certainly a sign that someone is no longer borderline. This phase's conclusion is marked by the patient's fullness of life—investment and satisfaction from work and from relationships outside of therapy.

Psychotherapy's Role in the Overall Treatment of Borderline Personality Disorder

In more advanced phases of treatment (phases III–IV), the case management problems subside, and the psychodynamic psychotherapist can more comfortably assume responsibilities for residual management issues such as collaboration with group therapists or with families. Although psychotherapy is central to achieving long-term health objectives with borderline patients, it is increasingly apparent that it is only one part of the optimal treatment program. For example, it is very clear that the borderline patient's social rehabilitation needs (e.g., listening to criticism, sharing attention, impulse control) are better served by modalities, such as a partial hospital or group therapy, with more instruction, peer interaction, and social consequences. A behavioral therapy, dialectical behavior therapy, appears more effective in diminishing self-destructive behavior. It also seems clear that medications can ease subjective distress more easily than psychotherapy and may even facilitate being able to function within psychotherapies. Thus, the modern psychotherapist must respect the value of what other modalities offer and, in my opinion, be ready to strongly urge—sometimes even insist on—a patient's participation in those other modalities that offer obvious advantages. This can be difficult. The borderline patient will want more one-to-one sessions and typically will hope that a sufficiently exclusive relationship with a therapist (or other person) will offer a solution to all their problems. Therapists still unfortunately can share their patient's hope. More commonly, therapists can recognize the unlikelihood of such a solution but nonetheless feel obligated to respect the patient's wishes. In contrast, I believe psychotherapists should advise their patients why they believe another modality would benefit them and then persevere, working through the patient's resistance. Borderline patients, despite protestation, can understand and appreciate good reasons and good intentions. They will rarely overtly and consciously defy good advice—if the therapist has the conviction to persevere.

Psychotherapy is distinguished from other modalities by its potential for a secure attachment to develop in which basic interpersonal problems of trust and intimacy can be repaired. This process takes time, depending on extended corrective experiences that are gradually internalized. Psychotherapy also offers some unique learning opportunities, because a well-trained and bright therapist offers insights into motivations and the links of present habits or beliefs to one's personal development. This adds meaning to life and a narrative coherence to one's life history. These issues that distinguish long-term individual psychotherapy are not offered by other modalities.

Conclusion/Summary

It is difficult to do justice to the contributions of the many creative and wise clinicians who have pioneered the development of psychotherapy for borderline personality disorder. Although I began this review with apologies for what was recognized would be incomplete and selective, I am impressed by how much more specific and confident I was able to be than was possible for Kernberg (1982) in a similar review. Although empirically loyal readers will continue to be disturbed by this review's primary reliance on clinical experience, the conclusions represented here do reflect an ongoing process of new knowledge being acquired. The conclusions that persist have been pruned by having endured criticisms, debate, and the competing claims of other modalities.

Largely and I think notably absent from this review are two topics that have often dominated discussions of psychotherapy with borderline patients: countertransference and boundary violations. Both subjects constitute large parts of the enormous literature describing problems created by borderline patients for unsuspecting therapists. Such problems became the major reason for defining the borderline syndrome—so that clinicians would not initiate therapies that were destructive to their own and the patient's health. No more psychoanalysis for "pseudoneurotic" (allegedly truly schizophrenic) patients, no more multiplication of medications onto toxicity in pursuit of treatment-resistant atypical depressions, no more unstructured pity within milieu programs, and no more late-night appointments to solve the patient's loneliness. The widespread recognition of what distinguishes this form of psychopathology has forewarned clinicians. Knowledgeable clinicians now can anticipate the stresses and strains on themselves and on usual practices that borderline patients will bring to bear. Those clinicians who want to practice psychotherapy with borderline patients can anticipate the countertransference problems and the complexities of managing boundary problems. Moreover, as emphasized in this review, it is now common, and I think advantageously so, that during the early phases of treatment psychotherapists do not work in isolation. This both provides monitors to oversights or excesses, should they occur, and diminishes the likelihood of such problems by containing splits or projections and flight. Finally, the increased awareness that clinicians require experience and training before they undertake psychotherapies—especially intensive therapies—is a major step toward delimiting countertransference and boundary failures.

I expect that our knowledge about individual psychotherapies will continue to grow slowly, incrementally adding refinements and certainty to what is believed and practiced. Current and future research projects will increasingly assist this knowledge base. But rather than adding new ideas or techniques, empirical research will primarily help resolve competing clinical claims that have developed and gained committed practitioners within the still robust clinical psychotherapeutic community. More impressive will be changes in thinking about psychotherapy that, already under way, are pushed by theory, economic forces, and the prevailing treatment paradigms. For example, psychotherapy is already being divided into competing types (dynamic vs. cognitive), and the distinguishing features of this modality will continue to be identified by observing how it interacts with (as opposed to contrasts with) activities such as case management. Even more clear is that psychotherapy with borderline patients will be seen as having phases during which the primary issues to be addressed will require different and increasingly specifiable types of interventions or techniques or responses from psychotherapists. This development of more specific sequences of problems and interventions will lend itself to more discrete empirical examinations.

There is no foreseeable risk that individual psychodynamic psychotherapy will become obsolete for borderline patients. The aspects of what it offers that have been distinctive (as noted, a connective attachment and a meaningful coherent narrative to one's life history) are not yet challenged by competitive strategies that can claim the same goals.

References

Adler G: The myth of the alliance with borderline patients. Am J Psychiatry 136:642–645, 1979

Adler G: Borderline Psychopathology and Its Therapy. New York, Jason Aronson, 1985

Akhtar S: Broken Structures: Severe Personality Disorders and Their Treatment. Northvale, NJ, Jason Aronson, 1982

Allen JG, Gabbard GO, Newson GE, et al: Detecting change in patient's collaboration within individual psychotherapy sessions. Psychotherapy 27:522–530, 1990

Bateman A, Fonagy P: The effectiveness of partial hospitalization in the treatment of borderline personality disorder—a randomized-controlled trial. Am J Psychiatry 156:1563–1569, 1999

Bender DS, Dolan RT, Skodol AE, et al: Treatment utilization by patients with personality disorders. (submitted)

Benjamin LS: Interpersonal Diagnosis and Treatment of Personality Disorders. New York, Guilford, 1993

Berkowitz CB, Gunderson JG, Smith GW: Psychoeducational multiple family treatment of borderline personality disorder, in The Multifamily Group. Edited by McFarlane WR. New York, Oxford University Press, 2000, pp 593–613

Fonagy P, Target M: Playing with reality, I: theory of mind and the normal development of psychic reality. Int J Psychoanal 77:217–233, 1996

Freidman H: Psychotherapy of borderline patients: the influence of theory on technique. Am J Psychiatry 132:1048–1052, 1975

Gabbard GO, Gunderson JG: Making the case for psychoanalytic therapies in the current psychiatric environment. J Am Psychoanal Assoc 47(2):679–740, 1999

Gabbard GO, Horwitz L, Frieswyk SH, et al: The effect of therapist interventions on the therapeutic alliance with borderline patients. J Am Psychoanal Assoc 36:697–727, 1988

Gabbard GO, Horwitz L, Allen JG, et al: Transference interpretation in the psychotherapy of borderline patients: a high-risk, high-gain phenomenon. Harv Rev Psychiatry 2:59–69, 1994

Greenspan ST, Sharfstein SS: Efficacy of psychotherapy: asking the right questions. Arch Gen Psychiatry 38:1213–1219, 1981

Gunderson JG: Borderline Personality Disorder. Washington, DC, American Psychiatric Press, 1984

Gunderson JG: The borderline patient's intolerance of aloneness: insecure attachments and therapist availability. Am J Psychiatry 153:752–758, 1996

Gunderson JG: Treatment of Borderline Personality Disorder. Washington, DC, American Psychiatric Press (in press)

Gunderson JG, Chu JA: Treatment implications of past trauma in borderline personality disorder. Harv Rev Psychiatry 1:75–81, 1993

Gunderson JG, Gabbard GO: Making the case for psychoanalytic therapies in the current psychiatric environment. JAPA 47(3):695, 1999

Gunderson JG, Frank AF, Ronningstam EF, et al: Early discontinuance of borderline patients from psychotherapy. J Nerv Ment Dis 177:38–42, 1989

Gunderson JG, Waldinger R, Sabo AN: Stages of change in dynamic psychotherapy with borderline patients: clinical and research implications. Psychotherapy Practice and Research 2:64–72, 1993

Gunderson JG, Najavits LM, Leonhard C, et al: Ontogeny of the therapeutic alliance in borderline patients. Psychotherapy Research 7:301–309, 1997

Horwitz L: Clinical Predictions in Psychotherapy. New York, Jason Aronson, 1974

Horwitz L, Gabbard G, Allen JG, et al: Borderline Personality Disorder: Tailoring the Psychotherapy to the Patient. Washington, DC, American Psychiatric Press, 1996

Kernberg OF: The treatment of patients with borderline personality organization. Int J Psychoanal 49:600–619, 1968

Kernberg OF: The psychotherapeutic treatment of borderline personalities, in Psychiatry 1982: The American Psychiatric Association Annual Review, Vol 1. Edited by Grinspoon L. Washington, DC, American Psychiatric Press, 1982, pp 470–486

Kernberg OF, Burstein E, Coyne L, et al: Final report of the Menninger Foundation's psychotherapy research project: psychotherapy and psychoanalysis. Bull Menninger Clin 34:1–2, 1972

Kernberg OF, Selzer MA, Koenigsberg HW, et al: Psychodynamic Psychotherapy of Borderline Patients. New York, Basic Books, 1989

Kopta SM, Howard KI, Lowry JL, et al: Patterns of symptomatic recovery in psychotherapy. J Consult Clin Psychol 62:1009–1016, 1994

Lanktree CB, Briere J: Outcome of therapy for sexually abused children: a repeated measures study. Child Abuse Negl 19:1145–1155, 1995

Linehan MM: Cognitive Behavioral Treatment of Borderline Personality Disorder. New York, Guilford, 1993

Linehan MM: Special feature: theory and treatment development and evaluation: reflections on Benjamin's "models for treatment." J Personal Disord 11:325–335, 1997

Linehan MM, Armstrong HE, Suarez A, et al: Cognitive-behavioral treatment of chronically parasuicidal borderline patients. Arch Gen Psychiatry 48:1016–1064, 1991

Luborsky L: Helping alliances in psychotherapy, in Successful Psychotherapy. Edited by Claghorn JL. New York, Brunner/Mazel, 1976, pp 92–116

Main T: The ailment. Br J Med Psychol 30:129–145, 1957

Masterson J: Treatment of the adolescent with borderline syndrome (a problem in separation-individuation). Bull Menninger Clin 35:5–18, 1971

Masterson J: Treatment of the Borderline Adolescent: A Developmental Approach. New York, John Wiley & Sons, 1972

Perry JC, Herman JC, Vanderkolk BA, et al: Psychotherapy and psychological trauma in borderline personality disorder. Psychoanalytic Annals 20:33–43, 1990

Pfohl B: A survey of attitudes about borderline personality disorder by discipline, clinical site, and geographic region. Unpublished manuscript, 1999

Selzer MA, Koenigsberg HW, Kernberg OF: The initial contract in the treatment of borderline patients. Am J Psychiatry 144:924–930, 1987

Skodol A, Buckley P, Charles E: Is there a characteristic pattern to the treatment history of clinical outpatients with borderline personality. J Nerv Ment Dis 171:405–410, 1983

Stevenson J, Meares R: An outcome study of psychotherapy for patients with borderline personality disorder. Am J Psychiatry 149:358–362, 1992

Swenson C: Kernberg and Linehan: two approaches to the borderline patient. J Personal Disord 311:26–35, 1989

Waldinger RJ, Gunderson JG: Completed psychotherapy with borderline patients. Am J Psychotherapy 38:190–202, 1984

Waldinger RJ, Gunderson JG: Effective Psychotherapy With Borderline Patients: Case Studies. Washington, DC, American Psychiatric Press, 1989

Wallerstein RS: Forty-Two Lives in Treatment: A Study of Psychoanalysis and Psychotherapy. New York, Guilford, 1986

Winnicott D: Transitional objects and transitional phenomena. Int J Psychoanal 34:89–97, 1953

Yeomans F, Selzer M, Clarkin J: Treating the Borderline Patient: A Contract-Based Approach. New York, Basic Books, 1992

Yeomans F, Selzer M, Clarkin J: Studying the treatment contract in intensive psychotherapy with borderline patients. Psychiatry 56:254–267, 1993

Zetzel E: A developmental approach to the borderline patient. Am J Psychiatry 128:867–871, 1971

Chapter 3

Combining Medication With Psychotherapy in the Treatment of Personality Disorders

Glen O. Gabbard, M.D.

Many personality disorders are currently being treated with a combination of medication and psychotherapy. Much of this practice is based on clinical impressions that some patients with personality disorders seem to have better outcomes with the combination than with either treatment alone. Empirical research support for this combination is quite limited. As suggested in other chapters in this volume, a growing literature on outcome supports the efficacy and effectiveness of psychotherapy for some personality disorders (Alden 1989; Bateman and Fonagy 1999; Cappe and Alden 1986; Gabbard 1997; Linehan et al. 1991; Meares et al. 1999; Stevenson and Meares 1992; Winston et al. 1994; Woody et al. 1985). Similarly, studies of the efficacy of psychopharmacological agents in the treatment of personality disorders have been published in increasing numbers over the last two decades (Coccaro 1993; Coccaro and Kavoussi 1997; Cowdry and Gardner 1988; Gabbard 1998; Kapfhammer and Hippius 1998; Markovitz 1995; Salzman et al. 1995; Soloff 1998).

Virtually no research exists that tests one modality alone versus combined pharmacotherapy and psychotherapy in the treatment of Axis II conditions. However, careful examination of the studies of psychotherapy reveals that numerous patients in those studies also were receiving medication. In addition, many of the pharmacotherapy trials involved patients who were receiving psychotherapy for their personality disorders while they were assigned to either placebo or an active agent. Hence, we must conclude that some of the studies designed to test a psychotherapeutic or pharmacotherapeutic modality actually were measuring outcomes of *combined* treatments for some patients.

In this chapter, I present a clinical rationale for the combination of pharmacotherapy and psychotherapy in personality disorders. I also discuss some of the problems and complications frequently encountered in combined treatment. Finally, I view the risk management and liability issues that should be taken into account when these two treatment components are used in the same patient.

Clinical Rationale for Combined Treatment

Many clinicians who add medications to an ongoing psychotherapy process with a personality disorder patient have given little thought to the conceptual basis of the combination. In fact, because personality disorders are notoriously difficult to treat, medications are often added out of a sense of countertransference despair rather than a carefully tailored treatment plan designed to address specific symptomatology. Several authors (Cloninger et al. 1993; Gabbard 1998, 1999, 2000; Gunderson and Links 1995; Koenigsberg 1992, 1994; Links et al. 1998; Soloff 1998) have outlined conceptual models that provide a rationale for using psychopharmacological agents in conjunction with psychotherapy. Borrowing from several of these models, I present an integrative rationale that incorporates our contemporary understanding of the nature of personality. Elsewhere (Gabbard, in press), I have outlined a conceptualization of personality disorders that is both biologically informed and psychodynamically based. Within this model, we can conceptualize four basic components of personality: 1) a genetically based biological temperament, 2) a constellation of internal object relations units that are linked to affect states and externalized in interpersonal relationships, 3) a characteristic set of defense mechanisms, and 4) a related cognitive style.

This integrative model can be used to conceptualize three roles that medications may play in the treatment of personality disorders: 1) they may modify temperament, 2) they may address specific target symptoms, and 3) they may treat comorbid Axis I disorders. These three strategies are here arbitrarily dissociated from one another, but in the clinical setting, these three domains overlap extensively. For the sake of clarity, I discuss each of them separately. As will soon become apparent, these domains and the treatment strategies connected to them have more empirical support for some personality disorders than for others.

Before we embark on this discussion, however, one point about combined treatment is essential. At best, medications should be considered useful adjuncts to psychotherapy in patients with personality disorders. No agent will effectively treat a personality disorder without associated psychotherapeutic intervention.

Temperament and Character

Cloninger et al. (1993) constructed a psychobiological model of personality that involves four dimensions of temperament and three dimensions of character (see Figure 3–1).

Within this model, approximately 50% of personality can be attributed to temperament, which is heavily influenced by genetic variables, and approximately 50% involves character traits that are only weakly affected by genetic factors and are predominantly accounted for by environmental variables.

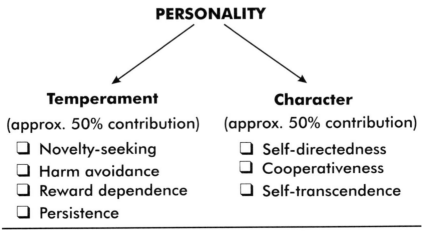

PERSONALITY

Temperament
(approx. 50% contribution)
❏ Novelty-seeking
❏ Harm avoidance
❏ Reward dependence
❏ Persistence

Character
(approx. 50% contribution)
❏ Self-directedness
❏ Cooperativeness
❏ Self-transcendence

Figure 3–1. A psychobiological model of personality.

The four dimensions of temperament are 1) novelty-seeking, characterized by frequent exploratory activity in response to novelty, impulsive decision making, extravagance in the approach to cues and reward, quick loss of temper, and active avoidance of frustration; 2) harm avoidance, which involves pessimistic worry about the future, avoidant behavior such as fear of uncertainty and shyness regarding strangers, and rapid fatigability; 3) reward dependence, characterized by sentimentality, social attachment, and dependence on the approval of others; and 4) persistence, which refers to the capacity for perseverance despite frustration and fatigue. These dimensions are 50%–60% heritable (independently of one another), manifest themselves early in life, and tend to persist throughout the life cycle.

Certain temperaments are characteristic of specific types of personality disorders. Cluster A personality disorders are strongly associated with low reward dependence. Cluster B patients tend to be high in novelty-seeking. Cluster C patients are high in harm avoidance. Patients with borderline personality disorder are unique in being high in *both* novelty-seeking and harm avoidance.

The three dimensions of character are shaped by family and social influences, trauma, and environmental stressors. Self-directedness involves acceptance of responsibility for one's choices rather than blaming others, acceptance of self, resourcefulness, and the identification of life goals and purposes. Cooperativeness is a measure of object relatedness and taps dimensions such as empathy, helpfulness, compassion, and social acceptance. Self-transcendence refers to the individual's spiritual acceptance, identifications beyond the self, and altruistic pursuits.

Cloninger and colleagues (1993) found that the character dimensions of self-directedness and cooperativeness are critical factors in the diagnosis of personality disorder. In fact, low self-directedness and low cooperativeness are associated with all categories of personality disorder. Whereas temperament is highly stable over time, even with psychotherapy, character is malleable and develops throughout adulthood (Svrakic et al. 1993).

This classification is somewhat controversial in that not all studies in behavioral genetics fully support this particular distinction between temperament and character. Moreover, character and temperament are inextricably intertwined in the clinical setting. Nevertheless, the model is of considerable heuristic value because it reminds the psychotherapist of the need to distinguish which features of personality are likely to respond to psychotherapy and which are not. A central point emphasized by Cloninger et al. (1993) is that the distinction between temperament and character may be essential for effective treatment: "Models that confound temperament and character may lead to therapeutic nihilism because they neglect distinctions crucial for effective treatment" (Svrakic et al. 1993, p. 999).

The character dimensions in this model readily lend themselves to more typical conceptual terms used by psychodynamic therapists. Specifically, the self-directedness dimension is closely linked to the psychoanalytic constructs of self-esteem, self-cohesion, self-representations, and ego functions, whereas cooperativeness is easily translatable into internal object relations as they are externalized and manifested in the interpersonal relationships of the individual. Self-transcendence, although less relevant to personality disorders, reflects certain mature defenses such as sublimation and altruism. Thus, medication may be useful to treat the temperament portion of the personality, whereas psychotherapy addresses the self-domain and the patient's internal object relations as they appear in the patient's narrative of other relationships and in the here-and-now transference–countertransference dimensions of the interaction with the therapist. Defenses and the associated cognitive style also may be useful foci of psychotherapy, although research has yet to distinguish in any systematic way which defenses are primarily genetic and part of temperament and which are shaped by interactions in the environment and are predominantly character (Gunderson et al. 1999; Marcus 1990). Some clinicians (Marcus 1990) have noted that antidepressant medications may decrease the rigidity of defenses and enhance the patient's observing ego capacity.

One clear implication of this distinction between temperament and character is that medications and psychotherapy may work synergistically in patients who have severe personality disorders.

Medications such as the selective serotonin reuptake inhibitors (SSRIs) and lithium may modify temperamental variables such as impulsivity, temper outbursts, and unmodulated anger, but they may be less helpful with self-concepts or the patient's basic internal object relationships. Patients with borderline personality disorder, for example, may respond to fluoxetine with decreases in anger and impulsivity (Coccaro and Kavoussi 1997; Markovitz 1995; Salzman et al. 1995), which may allow them to be more reflective and thoughtful about what is transpiring between the patient and the therapist.

> Mr. A, a 28-year-old man with borderline personality disorder, constantly complained that his therapist was not helping him. In one session, he said to his therapist, "It seems like I have to do all the work here. I wish you'd tell me what was wrong and what I need to do about it. I don't know if you're even competent to treat someone like me. I can't even tell if you really know what you're doing."
>
> The therapist responded, "When I *do* say something, you tend to say that it's unhelpful or stupid."
>
> The patient then exploded in anger and screamed at the therapist, "That's because it *is* stupid! You try to make it my problem that I see your comments as incompetent! I should try to find a therapist who actually knows what he's doing."
>
> Despite this threat, Mr. A continued to see his therapist and, after approximately 4 weeks on fluoxetine, began to show changes in his capacity to collaborate with the therapist on what was happening in the process. The therapist pointed out to the patient that he seemed better able to tolerate the therapist's observations and think about them a bit.
>
> The patient replied in a calm and measured voice, "I know I have a short fuse. I think I get angry with you because I'm so frustrated that nothing seems to change in my life. I know you're trying to help me, but I wish you'd do more and do it faster."
>
> In this breakthrough, Mr. A's usual anger was remarkably absent. The affective "background noise" was reduced by the fluoxetine, so the patient became more reflective and able to think about his own contribution to the difficulties in the therapeutic relationship. His basic mode of object relatedness was not greatly altered, but he was able to think about it in a way that was more constructive for the psychotherapy.

Target Symptoms

Because of the difficulty inherent in treating personality disorders, the assessment of the outcome of any particular intervention may be extraordinarily complicated. The placebo response rate in Axis II conditions such as borderline personality disorder is high (Salzman et al. 1995; Soloff et al. 1993), and almost any agent may make the patient feel globally better for a while. Many psychopharmacologists argue that clinicians should target a particular symptom and have reasonably clear means of measuring whether the symptom has responded to the agent prescribed (Links et al. 1998; Siever and Davis 1991; Soloff 1998). Hence, pharmacotherapy for personality disorders is generally approached from the standpoint of specific symptoms or symptom clusters that are targeted by specific agents (Gabbard 1998; Gunderson and Links 1995; Kapfhammer and Hippius 1998; Links et al. 1998; Soloff 1998). To be sure, this strategy is not a panacea because several medications have broad and nonspecific effects when treating personality disorders (Coccaro 1993; Links et al. 1998). For example, in a 14-week double-blind, placebo-controlled trial in 31 patients with borderline personality disorder, Markovitz (1995) found far-ranging improvements in the fluoxetine-treated group compared with the placebo-treated group. The group receiving fluoxetine showed significant positive changes in depression, anxiety, paranoia, psychoticism, interpersonal sensitivity, obsessionality, and hostility as well as in global functioning.

Despite this "wide scatter" approach of several drugs commonly used to treat personality disorders, dividing symptoms into clusters that may respond to particular medications is a way of ordering the chaos of personality disorder treatment and systematically thinking through the rationale for each agent prescribed. Soloff (1998), for example, developed a tentative algorithm based on three symptomatic clusters: cognitive-perceptual, impulsive-behavioral, and affective. These symptom domains are based on a dimensional understanding of personality that transcends the usual definitions of Axis I and Axis II disorders. Soloff acknowledged that an algorithm based on rigorous randomized, controlled trials for every agent is not yet possible, but he provided clinical guidelines that may be useful for psychiatrists who are feeling overwhelmed by a plethora of symptomatic expressions in a particular patient. One advantage of this target symptom approach is that it recognizes that different manifestations of personality disorder require different pharmacotherapeutic strategies. In other words, we do not speak in terms of "the treatment of choice" for conditions such as borderline personality disorder. Rather, we consider questions such as "which agent works best for which borderline patient with which symptomatic expression?"

Cognitive-Perceptual Symptoms

Symptoms such as brief psychotic episodes characterized by paranoid ideation and ideas of reference, depersonalization, derealization, and various subtle forms of thought disorder may be encountered in Cluster A personality disorders, such as schizotypal and paranoid personality disorders, and in Cluster B conditions, such as borderline personality disorder. Low-dose conventional neuroleptics have proven to be useful in these patients (Cowdry and Gardner 1988; S. E. Goldberg et al. 1986; Serban and Siegel 1984; Soloff et al. 1986, 1989). The various traditional neuroleptics that have been tried have comparable efficacy and are generally superior to placebo in most trials. As expected, they have been shown to improve perceptual and cognitive symptoms, but they also occasionally improve other symptoms, such as anxiety and depression.

Because of the risk of tardive dyskinesia with conventional neuroleptics, many clinicians now use atypical neuroleptics as first-line agents. Randomized, placebo-controlled trials are being conducted, but data to guide the clinician are limited at this point. Nevertheless, open-label trials have been promising (Benedetti et al. 1998; Frankenburg and Zanarini 1993), and these medications should be considered along with the traditional neuroleptics. Finally, the 1995 Markovitz study mentioned earlier in this chapter noted some improvement in cognitive and perceptual symptoms from high doses (80 mg/day) of fluoxetine, so SSRIs also may be considered in conjunction with neuroleptics for this symptom cluster.

Impulsive-Behavioral Symptoms

In the impulsive-behavioral symptom domain, explosive temper tantrums, reckless behavior, low frustration tolerance, verbal or physical aggression, recurrent suicidal threats, self-mutilation, and binges with food, sex, spending, or substance abuse are found. These symptoms commonly occur in Cluster B personality disorders, and double-blind, placebo-controlled trials suggest that an SSRI is probably the first-line agent (Coccaro and Kavoussi 1997; Markovitz 1995; Salzman et al. 1995).

Soloff (1998) recommended in his algorithm to add a low-dose neuroleptic if these impulsive behaviors are not sufficiently reduced by an SSRI. If the patient continues to be unresponsive, the clinician can consider adding lithium carbonate or switching to a monoamine oxidase inhibitor (MAOI). Obviously, psychiatrists who prescribe MAOIs must do so with considerable caution because patients with borderline personality disorder are notoriously noncompliant with treatment regimens, and a special diet is required to avoid life-threatening side effects when a patient is taking an MAOI. The therapeutic alliance with the patient must be sufficiently sound and well established so that the patient can be counted on to talk about going off the diet before acting impulsively.

When explosiveness or impulsivity continue after a trial on the previous medications, carbamazepine or divalproex can be considered. Both must be regarded as experimental because there is little evidence for their effectiveness. One double-blind, crossover study (Cowdry and Gardner 1988) reported that carbamazepine was effective in reducing behavioral dyscontrol in patients with borderline personality disorder. Similarly, in a preliminary report on a 10-week double-blind, placebo-controlled trial of divalproex (Hollander 1999), patients taking divalproex showed global improvements that were not characteristic of the placebo group. Divalproex-treated patients also improved on one aggression scale (but not the other) and showed improvements in depression as well. Finally, atypical neuroleptics may be considered as a last resort.

When self-mutilation behaviors do not respond to SSRIs or other agents, clinicians may want to consider naltrexone in patients with borderline personality disorder, even though the evidence supporting the use of this agent is far from rigorous. In an open-label trial, Roth et al. (1996) gave 50 mg/day of naltrexone to seven female borderline patients with self-harm behavior. Within a mean follow-up of 10.7 weeks, six of the seven patients had totally eliminated the self-harm behavior. The investigators concluded that naltrexone might be useful for patients who engage in self-mutilating behavior accompanied by a reduction in dysphoria and analgesia. Links et al. (1998) stressed that because of the demonstrated effectiveness of naltrexone in assisting patients to remain abstinent from alcohol, this agent may be of particular benefit with self-mutilating patients who also have substance abuse problems.

Controlled studies have shown that patients with borderline and other severe personality disorders who do not have comorbid affective disorders nevertheless improve with the administration of fluoxetine (Coccaro and Kavoussi 1997; Markovitz 1995). Moreover, tricyclic antidepressants have been shown to be of limited or no value in the treatment of borderline personality disorder (Soloff 1998). In some patients, symptoms may even worsen while taking tricyclic antidepressants. Hence, there appears to be an affective dysregulation that is emblematic of some personality disorders and differs from Axis I affective disorder (this distinction will be elaborated on in the subsequent section). When one SSRI does not appear to be effective, it is reasonable to switch to another SSRI with the expectation that some patients who do not respond to the first will respond to the second. Limited data from uncontrolled studies suggest that SSRIs that act on multiple transmitters, such as nefazodone or venlafaxine, may be effective when a pure SSRI is not. Markovitz (1995) also suggested that pushing these agents into a high dosage range may be necessary before optimal response is obtained.

If the affective dysregulation symptoms are not responsive to an SSRI, Soloff (1998) suggested trying a low-dose anxiolytic such as clonazepam if anxiety is present and a low-dose neuroleptic if anger is present. Alprazolam should be avoided because it tends to produce rather serious disinhibition in borderline personality disorder patients (Cowdry and Gardner 1988). Clonazepam does not seem to produce the same problematic reaction. In addition, clonazepam increases the availability of serotonin, which may account for its usefulness as an augmenting agent with an SSRI.

Soloff suggested that if the symptoms of affective dysregulation still do not respond, they can be treated next by a switch to an MAOI. This family of medications may help to improve angry affects and impulse control (Cowdry and Gardner 1988; Liebowitz et al. 1988). The same caveats noted in the discussion of impulsive-behavioral symptoms apply to this cluster as well. Finally, lithium can be considered as a last strategy, although the data and support for its use as a stabilizer of affective dysregulation symptoms in personality disorders are quite limited.

Affective Symptoms

Having summarized the three different symptom clusters and the medication strategies associated with them, we must keep in mind that these symptom domains can become blurred in the clinical situation. M. Zanarini (personal communication, July 1999) found in a follow-up study of borderline patients that the average patient was taking 3.5 medications, suggesting that in the real world, the target-symptom approach may get lost in the shuffle. Clinicians can best measure outcome by tying their assessment to specific behavioral changes that are targeted. In addition, virtually no literature exists on the use of any of these agents in the maintenance phase of personality disorders. The decision to continue medication after the acute symptomatic picture improves is a trial-and-error endeavor without clear guidelines. Many experienced clinicians have noted anecdotally that the so-called poop-out effect of SSRIs is frequently noted in personality disorder patients as well. This effect may be obscured by the fact that many personality disorder patients respond positively when the agent is initially introduced, perhaps in part because of placebo effects, and when the "honeymoon" phase wears off, they may feel quite disillusioned with the drug.

This review of the literature on treating target symptoms reflects the fact that most of the research has involved patients with borderline personality disorder. These strategies have been summarized in Table 3–1.

Table 3–1.   Medication strategies for borderline personality disorder target symptoms

Cognitive-perceptual symptoms	Impulsive-behavioral symptoms	Affective dysregulation symptoms
Low-dose traditional neuroleptic	SSRI	SSRI
Atypical neuroleptic	Low-dose neuroleptic	Low-dose neuroleptic
SSRI	Lithium carbonate	Clonazepam[a]
	MAOI[b]	MAOI[b]
	Carbamazepine	Lithium
	Divalproex	
	Atypical neuroleptic	
	Naltrexone (if self-mutilation and/or alcohol abuse are present)	

Note.   MAOI = monoamine oxidase inhibitor; SSRI = selective serotonin reuptake inhibitor.
[a]Do not use alprazolam because it may result in disinhibition.
[b]Should be used with considerable caution because of dietary restrictions.

Comorbid Axis I Conditions

It has long been known that there is a high rate of comorbidity between personality disorders and depression. Rates of comorbid depression in borderline personality disorder range from 24% to 87% (Docherty et al. 1986; Jonas and Pope 1992), and comorbidity rates for depressive illness are similar for other personality disorders as well (Tyrer et al. 1997). Even in a nonpatient sample (Zimmerman and Coryell 1989), 38.5% of the subjects with personality disorder diagnoses had a history of major depression.

It is also reasonably well established that patients with depression and comorbid personality disorders have poorer treatment responses than depressed patients without personality disorders. Pfohl et al. (1984) reported that depressed patients with personality disorders have poorer social support, higher rates of separation and divorce, and more life stressors than depressed patients without personality disorders, all of which may make their treatment more complicated. Patients with personality disorders also may be noncompliant with treatment plans and find it more difficult to form a therapeutic alliance with their treaters (Shea et al. 1992). In addition, they may activate a variety of countertransference reactions in clinicians that may affect those clinicians' ability to conduct effective psychotherapy or use good judgment in prescribing (Gabbard 1998).

In keeping with the notion that depression in personality disorders may represent a distinct entity, another reason for poorer response may be that the depression in patients with personality disorders may have features different from those of the classic Axis I major depression. Gunderson and Philips (1991) and Rogers et al. (1995) distinguished between the characterological depression associated with borderline personality disorder and a more classic unipolar depression (see Table 3–2).

The depression of the borderline patient is often characterized by emptiness and feelings of neediness and anger. When the patient says, "I'm depressed," he or she may mean that no one is available to perform caregiving functions. This anaclitic tendency and the intense anger associated with the depression present quite a different clinical picture from that of the usual unipolar major depression. When tricyclic antidepressants were the first-line treatment for depression, many of these patients' symptoms did not respond or worsened. Now that SSRIs are first-line treatments for *both* borderline personality disorder and major depression, this distinction may not be as significant for choice of psychopharmacological agent. Because borderline patients who do not have comorbid Axis I major depression still respond to SSRIs (Coccaro and Kavoussi 1997; Markovitz 1995), this outcome suggests that SSRIs may treat an underlying temperament in borderline personality disorder rather than depression. Indeed, the neuroticism temperament, which is closely linked to the harm-avoidance temperament in the Cloninger et al. (1993) model, is common to both certain personality disorders and depression (Gunderson et al. 1999). These common

Table 3–2. Differential diagnosis of characterological depression typical of borderline personality disorder and major depressive disorder

Borderline characterological disorder	Shared characteristics	Major depressive disorder
Loneliness	Depressed mood: early onset, sustained	Guilt feelings, remorse
Emptiness	Worthlessness, hopelessness	Withdrawal/ agitation
Repeated suicidal gestures	Object hunger (without gestures)	Suicidality
Conscious rage	Dependency in relationships	Stable relationships
Demanding, hostile, dependent relationships	Fragile self-esteem	Concern with defeat, failures
Concern with interpersonal loss, separation		Caregiving welcomed (with history of independence)
Illusory self-sufficiency (with history of dependency)		More severe vegetative symptoms

Source. Based on Gunderson and Phillips 1991.

temperamental underpinnings suggest that certain treatment approaches might be effective for both conditions.

This discussion of the interface between affective disorder and personality disorder is a good example of why it is somewhat arbitrary to separate out three different pharmacotherapeutic strategies. Temperament, symptom clusters, and Axis I comorbid disorders are conceptually overlapping. Psychiatric problems observed in the clinical setting do not necessarily conform neatly to our methods of classifying and understanding psychiatric disorders. A similar problem occurs when an Axis I disorder is operationally almost indistinguishable from an Axis II condition. Such is the case with generalized social phobia and avoidant personality disorder.

Several studies involving medication trials for social phobia have found that as the symptoms of this Axis I disorder improve, the traits of avoidant personality disorder are also reduced (Links et al. 1998). Liebowitz et al. (1992) found that avoidant personality features in patients who received diagnoses of social phobia were responsive to phenelzine. When social phobia was treated with moclobemide and phenelzine (Versiani et al. 1992), there was a marked difference between medication-treated patients and placebo-treated patients when the criteria for avoidant personality disorder were examined. After 8 weeks of treatment, only 3 of the 27 patients receiving one of the active medications still met criteria for avoidant personality disorder, whereas 14 of the 16 in the placebo group still met criteria. Recent evidence (Stein et al. 1998) that paroxetine and possibly other SSRIs are effective in treating generalized social phobia suggests that avoidant personality disorder traits also may respond to those agents.

This example of the treatment of social phobia shows how pharmacological treatment of an Axis I disorder may lead to resolution of an Axis II condition (Links et al. 1998). A common underlying temperament may be at the heart of both conditions, and the modification of that temperament may lead to an improved capacity to use psychotherapy and take the risks necessary to confront feared situations. Gabbard and Bartlett (1998) have shown in a clinical example how the treatment of social phobia symptoms with an SSRI may confront a patient with his or her characterological reluctance to face a situation that is feared even when the anxiety symptoms are much improved.

Regardless of the conceptual complexities of distinguishing Axis I from Axis II disorders, most experts would agree that the treatment of Axis I disorders in patients with personality disorders should be a very high priority for psychopharmacological intervention (Links et al. 1998). In a long-term follow-up study of borderline patients, Stone (1990) noted that patients who had comorbid affective disorder and untreated alcoholism had a very high suicide rate, and he suggested that the treatment of these Axis I comorbid conditions should be the first priority in a comprehensive treatment plan.

Clinical Problems

When a personality disorder patient in psychotherapy is started on a carefully chosen psychotropic medication, several clinical considerations make the treatment complex. Many of these complexities can be examined in the context of the two models commonly used in clinical practice to combine pharmacotherapy and psychotherapy. The one-person model involves a psychiatrist who both conducts the psychotherapy and prescribes the medication for the same patient at the same time. The two-person model divides these functions so that one clinician prescribes the medication and another conducts the psychotherapy.

One-Person Model

Psychiatry as a medical specialty is designed to be integrative. The psychiatrist is trained to examine biological, psychological, and social/cultural factors in the etiology of psychiatric illness and in the planning of a comprehensive treatment. Hence, a psychiatrist is in a unique position among mental health professionals to be able to conduct both treatments. If the psychiatrist feels adequately trained in both modalities, the one-person model has particular advantages. All transferences, countertransferences, and resistances are dealt with by one clinician. The one-person model avoids the fragmentation and splitting so typical of the two-person model. Another advantage is that compliance problems with the medication can be examined directly in the context of the specific transferences that are developing in the psychotherapy and the clinician's intimate knowledge of the patient's internal object relations.

Poor treatment adherence is characteristic of patients with personality disorders (Links et al. 1998). Patients with borderline personality disorder have been studied most thoroughly. In one prospective study of 60 inpatients with borderline personality disorder referred for psychotherapy, 43% of the patients failed to complete 6 months of treatment (Gunderson et al. 1989). From 40% to 60% of patients with borderline personality disorder in psychopharmacology studies drop out of treatment before the study is completed (Cowdry and Gardner 1988; Links et al. 1990).

The addition of a medication such as an SSRI may reduce anger and thus improve the therapeutic alliance in the psychotherapy, whereas the psychotherapeutic exploration may help the patient understand any negative meanings of the medication that may lead to noncompliance with the agent that has been prescribed.

Because SSRIs are commonly prescribed to patients with severe personality disorders, sexual side effects may play a role in the patients' noncompliance. Sexual anxieties and a thorough sense of shame about sexuality may prevent patients with these side effects from discussing them openly with a psychopharmacologist they see for 15 minutes every few months. On the other hand, if some degree of trust is established with a psychotherapist seen weekly, patients may be able to talk about the side effects forthrightly rather than secretly discontinue the medication because of their embarrassment.

A common development in combined treatment is transference to the medication itself (Adelman 1985; Gabbard 2000; Waldinger and Frank 1989). This phenomenon may work to the treatment's advantage when the pill serves as a transitional object that symbolically represents the therapist. With borderline personality disorder patients who have poorly developed object constancy, the pill may serve as a substitute for the therapist while he or she is on vacation and soothe the patient's feeling of abandonment. Other transference reactions to the medication may facilitate the working through of the patient's internal object relations, as in the following example:

> Ms. B, a 31-year-old patient with borderline personality disorder, had been in psychotherapy for 7 months when her therapist first prescribed fluoxetine because of her problems with affective dysregulation and feeling empty and unloved. The patient was thrilled with the therapist's decision to prescribe, and she told the therapist, "I can't tell you how happy I am that you finally agreed to this. My friend Marjorie said that Prozac has been the most helpful thing in her whole treatment. I didn't tell you this, but about 2 weeks ago, I actually took one of her capsules just to see how it would feel. I knew you wouldn't approve, but I had to see for myself. It was amazing how much better I felt in just about 30 minutes. I knew then that it would have the same effect on me that it had on Marjorie."

The therapist replied, "I'm glad you were able to tell me that, because for us to work together collaboratively on the medication, I really have to depend on your complete openness and honesty. I won't be able to tell how the medication is doing unless you're completely candid."

Ms. B responded, "Okay, from now on I'll tell you what's going on with the medication. I just thought you'd disapprove of my taking it without discussing it with you."

The therapist replied, "Well, I *do* think it's better if we talk about any medication decision, but I think I'd be more likely to be disapproving if you concealed what you're doing with medication. The other thing I want to stress is that I think you're setting yourself up by thinking that the medication is going to be a panacea of sorts. There's nothing magical about Prozac. We should expect rather modest results. You may feel a little less depressed and a little less angry, and if it works, we may be able to deal with your problems in psychotherapy more effectively. It won't be a cure, and your problems will remain." Ms. B appeared to accept the therapist's cautionary note and started the medication the next day.

As expected, the patient initially felt that the fluoxetine was tremendously soothing and seemed much brighter in her therapy hours. However, this idealization of the medication began to crumble in a matter of weeks, and 2 months after starting the medication, she came to the therapy and said, "I have this other friend who's taking Effexor, and I was wondering if maybe I could switch to that."

The therapist asked why she wanted to change. Ms. B explained, "Well, it seemed to work at first, but now I feel like the same problems are returning. I can't seem to soothe myself when I'm alone on weekends. I feel depressed all the time. I don't feel like anyone really loves me. Why can't I try another pill?"

The therapist explained, "Before switching to another agent, we really need to push the dose up a bit further. You're taking only 40 mg, and some people don't respond until the dose is as high as 80 mg/day."

Ms. B angrily said, "I don't think you're listening to me. I don't want to take this any more. You used to be more sympathetic and understanding. Now I feel like you're practicing out of some textbook instead of listening to what I tell you I need."

This vignette illustrates several features of combining medication and psychotherapy in a borderline patient. First, the psychopharmacological agent becomes imbued with an idealized transference that crumbles over time. This transference to the fluoxetine parallels the transference to the therapist who is initially idealized and eventually seen as unhelpful and insensitive. Both the transference to the medication and the transference to the therapist reflect the patient's internal object relations that are enacted repeatedly in different situations—namely, an unrealistic expectation that an omnipotent other will magically take care of all the internal turmoil only to be disappointed when no magic ensues. The therapist continued to work with Ms. B to help her recognize that ultimately she would have to rely on her own resources to cope with her internal dysphoria. No panacea would come from outside, whether in the form of a therapist or a medication, and she would have to develop her internal coping capacities. Moreover, many patients, like Ms. B, have only a minimal response to SSRIs.

Borderline patients frequently manifest a sense of urgency in their requests of clinicians (Gabbard and Wilkinson 1994). Delay mechanisms may be poorly developed, so waiting to receive a medication may feel unbearable. Patients like Ms. B may experiment with various agents, and clinicians like Ms. B's therapist may feel pressured to prescribe before sufficient reflection on the indications and contraindications.

Another point illustrated by this vignette is that the therapist must introduce a new medication into the process by emphasizing the modest effects to be expected rather than overselling it to the patient. Also, when the therapist learns about the patient's episode of experimenting with a friend's medication, he does not respond with a punitive attitude but rather emphasizes the need for candor. The therapist must be wary of becoming a punitive object who is more concerned about policing than helping the patient.

Psychiatrists who are both prescribing medication and conducting psychotherapy are somewhat like physicists who simultaneously thinks in terms of waves and particles. In other words, psychiatrists have to consider neurotransmitters and vegetative symptoms while keeping in mind transference, resistance, and internal object relations. They must shift back and forth between an empathic–introspective subjective approach and a more objective descriptive approach (Gabbard 1999). The therapist may stress a more exploratory and collaborative approach when examining the patient's internal world, whereas a more didactic and authoritarian posture may be necessary when dealing with medication. The therapist may need to cite research on topics such as prevention of relapse through maintenance dosages. The psychotherapist may be encouraging the patient to talk rather than act, but the shift to the prescribing mode may emphasize clear and decisive action rather than reflection. This back-and-forth shift may be jarring to both clinician and patient. To make this transition more structured, some therapists will use a few minutes at the beginning or end of the session to talk about target symptoms and side effects as a way of assessing the effectiveness of the medication. Others will incorporate those questions in the context of the psychotherapy session. As illustrated in the vignette with Ms. B, however, the meaning of the medication to the patient always must be explored, and the therapist must avoid splitting off the medication as though it is not an integrative part of the psychotherapy.

Two-Person Model

In the two-person model, one clinician, usually a psychiatrist, prescribes the medication, and another clinician conducts the psychotherapy. Practical considerations often determine which model is used. For example, many psychiatrists who are skilled psychotherapists do not keep up with the psychopharmacology literature and do not feel competent to prescribe certain medications. The opposite situation also may contribute to the selection of the two-person model. If a psychopharmacologist who is seeing a patient to prescribe medication diagnoses a serious personality disorder, he or she may not feel experienced or knowledgeable about the psychotherapy for such patients and may wish to refer to another clinician for psychotherapy. Obviously, when psychotherapy is conducted by a nonmedical therapist, referral to a psychiatrist or another physician is required to prescribe medication.

In recent years in the United States, clinicians working in managed care settings may have little choice in the matter. Managed care reviewers may stipulate that psychotherapy must be conducted by a nonmedical therapist because they view it as less expensive than having a psychiatrist both conduct the psychotherapy and prescribe the medication. Psychiatrists are frequently limited to 15-minute medication checks. Whether this arrangement is less costly than having one clinician perform both functions has not actually been rigorously tested.

The two-person model may have some advantages in particular clinical situations (Waldinger and Frank 1989). The therapist may gain consultation from a colleague who is working from another perspective. The intensity of the transference may be diluted by having two treaters. In some cases, the two-person model may help because the patient cannot avoid psychotherapeutic issues by focusing on medication during the psychotherapy sessions.

On the other hand, the practice of having one person conduct the psychotherapy and another prescribe medication is a setup for splitting problems (Gabbard 1989, 1999; Waldinger and Frank 1989). A clinical example illustrates the common difficulties encountered:

> Ms. C had been in psychotherapy for 11 months when she was referred to Dr. D, a well-known psychopharmacology expert. She had borderline personality disorder, and her therapist hoped that her explosive outbursts of anger would be improved by medication. The psychopharmacologist evaluated her for 45 minutes and prescribed paroxetine.
>
> At her follow-up appointment with Dr. D, Ms. C told him that it was a relief to finally see a doctor who really listened to her and took her concerns seriously. She asked Dr. D if he knew her therapist, and Dr. D replied that he had met her but did not know her well. Ms. C went on, "I don't want to sound like I'm bad-mouthing her, but I don't know if she's really doing her job. Do you know what kind of reputation she has?"
>
> Dr. D replied that he was not familiar with her reputation. Ms. C continued, "Well, for 11 months she just sat there while I kept telling her I needed medication. A lot of the time she looked sleepy or like her attention was wandering. Do you think she should have waited 11 months before referring me for a medication evaluation?"
>
> Dr. D, who was not psychodynamically trained, began to get "sucked in" to the splitting process and responded, "Well, let

me put it this way. I would have had you on medication within 2 weeks if I'd been the main treater."

At her next therapy appointment, Ms. C told her therapist, "I'm starting to doubt if you're a competent practitioner. Dr. D told me that if he had been treating me, he would have started me on medication within the first 2 weeks of seeing me. You just sat there and waited and waited and waited."

Her therapist explained, "For a long time, it was unclear whether medication would help you."

Ms. C responded, "Now you're sounding defensive!"

The therapist retorted, "Of course I'm defensive. You're criticizing me behind my back to a colleague and trying to ruin my reputation."

At this point, Ms. C began to cry: "I can't believe you're attacking me like this. I'm just trying to get good care for myself, and all you can think about is you!"

This tendency for the prescribing doctor to become idealized while the therapist is devalued is a common development in the two-person model. The reverse is also common, in which the prescribing physician is seen as too rushed in his or her 15-minute medication check to listen to the patient and attend to the patient's needs. The therapist, by contrast, spends more time and may be viewed as more engaged. In either case, this scenario involves a combination of splitting and projective identification (Gabbard 1989, 1994). Ms. C, for example, projected an idealized object representation onto Dr. D and then treated him in such a way that he conformed to the idealized representation. By presenting herself as a grateful patient of Dr. D and a victim of her psychotherapist, Ms. C induced Dr. D to take on the role of the omnipotent rescuer who wanted to save her from the neglectful treatment she was receiving from her therapist. Similarly, Ms. C projected the devalued object representation onto her therapist and then made critical and disparaging comments that irritated her therapist sufficiently that she began to enact the "bad object" role by erupting in anger at her patients.

This type of splitting is inherent in borderline personality disorder and cannot be entirely prevented. Nevertheless, the prescriber and the psychotherapist can take several measures to avoid the kind of destructive process depicted in this vignette. First, it should be made clear to the patient that the two treaters are members of a treatment team who will consult with each other as needed. If the patient refuses to give permission for consultation between the two, the clinician probably should not agree to be involved in the treatment. In the absence of regular communication with a colleague, a clinician may easily take the patient's report at face value and collude with the patient in a global devaluation of what the other clinician is doing.

In many cases, communication does not occur because the time spent consulting with the other treater is not reimbursed by a third party or managed care company. Hence, such communication is often relegated to low priority in the clinician's list of things to do. In managed care settings, the psychotherapist and the pharmacotherapist are often thrown together in what Meyer and Simon (1999a) have called a "clinical shotgun wedding" (p. 244). Neither clinician particularly wants to collaborate with the other, but economic forces have demanded a split treatment situation resented by each member. The feelings around this arrangement may be acted out by not communicating.

Risk Management and Liability Issues in the Two-Person Model

As the two-person model has become increasingly common, a literature on risk management and liability issues has evolved (Appelbaum 1991; Bradley 1990; R. S. Goldberg et al. 1991; Meyer and Simon 1999a, 1999b; Sederer et al. 1998; Woodward et al. 1993). Many prescribing physicians have become painfully aware that patients can sue anyone involved in their treatment, no matter how peripheral that involvement is. Even though the pharmacotherapist may see the patient rarely while the psychotherapist appears to have the major clinical responsibility, attorneys involved in litigation are mainly interested in identifying who has the "deepest pockets." In some cases, the prescribing physician or the institution where the physician is employed may have deeper pockets than the nonmedical psychotherapist. In any combined treatment, clinicians should clarify whether the relationship is 1) *consultative,* in which a psychiatrist merely offers an opinion without assuming any responsibility for the patient's ongoing care; 2) *supervisory,* in which the psychiatrist is responsible for overseeing and directing all aspects of the patient's treatment, and the therapist is not authorized to act autonomously without supervision; or 3) *collaborative,* in which clinicians share responsibility and are professionally interdependent (Meyer and Simon 1999a). Psychiatrists must recognize that regardless of how infrequently they meet with a patient, their clinical responsibility cannot simply be delegated to the psychotherapist. In the collaborative arrangement, which is by far the most common, limited communication often leaves both clinicians with considerable ambiguity about who is responsible for what.

Patients with severe personality disorders frequently require a treatment team that involves more than one clinician. In any team situation, clear agreement about which clinician is assuming the primary overall responsibility for the patient's safety and treatment is necessary. This clinician is designated as the final authority on decisions about hospitalization, the introduction or discontinuation of a particular treatment modality, and the monitoring of safety. This person usually should be a psychiatrist because a considerable range of expertise and knowledge is necessary for this form of responsibility. In some settings, a mental health professional other than a psychiatrist takes on this responsibility. In either case, however, explicit discussion of several issues should take place at the beginning of the treatment (Meyer and Simon 1999b).

First, the clinicians involved should establish that each is competent to administer the treatment and that each has sufficient professional liability insurance. The patient should give explicit consent for the prescribing psychiatrist and the psychotherapist to talk about the treatment as needed. Specifically, the two clinicians should agree to inform each other when a significant change in the treatment is being contemplated. They should also decide who should be responsible for covering during vacations, who should take emergency calls that may require patient hospitalization on evenings or weekends, and who should communicate to outside parties, such as family, employers, or managed care reviewers.

In a collaborative, rather than consultative or supervisory, relationship, it should be made explicit that the prescribing psychiatrist is not responsible for supervising the psychotherapy by the nonmedical therapist. The two clinicians also should agree that when the patient begins to disparage one of the treaters, the clinician who receives that information should contact the other treater to discuss what is going on rather than to act on the information given by the patient. When the patient knows that the two treaters will discuss any accusations he or she makes about one of the clinicians, some of the splitting that is so typical in combined treatment is diffused.

Finally, there should be an understanding that either the prescribing physician or the psychotherapist can choose to terminate participation in the treatment if either feels that the collaboration is not working. Obviously, sufficient notice must be given so that a replacement for the departing clinician can be found. Before this measure is taken, it is often useful for treaters to meet with a consultant to see if they can find a way to work out their differences (Gabbard 1989).

Summary

Combined treatment has become the standard approach to the treatment of most personality disorders. The rationale for adding medication is generally based on the assumption that one is treating temperament, target symptoms of the Axis II condition itself, or comorbid Axis I disorders. Careful attention to the measurement of treatment goals is essential to avoid a polypharmacy approach based on countertransference exasperation. The meaning of medication should be assessed in the psychotherapy and viewed as an integral part of an overall treatment plan. Both one-person and two-person models of combining psychotherapy and pharmacotherapy may be useful, but various complications are common in both models. When multiple treaters are involved, liability and risk management issues must be considered and prevented through clear and regular communication between treaters.

References

Adelman SA: Pills as transitional objects: a dynamic understanding of the use of medication in psychotherapy. Psychiatry 48:246–253, 1985

Alden L: Short-term structured treatment for avoidant personality disorder. J Consult Clin Psychol 57:756–764, 1989

Appelbaum PS: General guidelines for psychiatrists who prescribe medication for patients treated by nonmedical psychotherapists. Hospital and Community Psychiatry 42:281–282, 1991

Bateman A, Fonagy P: The effectiveness of partial hospitalization in the treatment of borderline personality disorder—a randomized-controlled trial. Am J Psychiatry 156:1563–1569, 1999

Benedetti F, Sforzini L, Columbo C, et al: Low-dose clozapine in acute and continuation treatment of severe borderline personality disorder. J Clin Psychiatry 59:103–107, 1998

Bradley SS: Nonphysician psychotherapist–physician pharmacotherapist: a new model for concurrent treatment. Psychiatr Clin North Am 13:307–322, 1990

Cappe RF, Alden LE: A comparison of treatment strategies for clients functionally impaired by extreme shyness and social avoidance. J Consult Clin Psychol 54:796–801, 1986

Cloninger CR, Svrakic DM, Pryzbeck TR: A psychobiological model of temperament and character. Arch Gen Psychiatry 50:975–990, 1993

Coccaro EF: Psychopharmacological studies in patients with personality disorders: review and perspective. J Personal Disord 7 (suppl):181–192, 1993

Coccaro EF, Kavoussi RJ: Fluoxetine and impulsive-aggressive behavior in personality disordered subjects. Arch Gen Psychiatry 54:1081–1088, 1997

Cowdry R, Gardner DL: Pharmacotherapy of borderline personality disorder: alprazolam, carbamazepine, trifluoperazine, and tranylcypromine. Arch Gen Psychiatry 45:111–119, 1988

Docherty JP, Fiester SJ, Shea T: Syndrome diagnosis in personality disorder, in American Psychiatric Association Annual Review of Psychiatry, Vol 5. Edited by Frances AJ, Hales RE. Washington, DC, American Psychiatric Press, 1986, pp 315–355

Frankenburg FR, Zanarini MC: Clozapine treatment of borderline patients: a preliminary study. Compr Psychiatry 34:402–405, 1993

Gabbard GO: Splitting in hospital treatment. Am J Psychiatry 146:444–451, 1989

Gabbard GO: Treatment of borderline patients in a multiple-treater setting. Psychiatr Clin North Am 17:839–850, 1994

Gabbard GO: Psychotherapy of personality disorders. Journal of Practical Psychiatry and Behavioral Health 3:327–333, 1997

Gabbard GO: Treatment-resistant borderline personality disorder. Psychiatric Annals 28:651–656, 1998

Gabbard GO: Combined psychotherapy and pharmacotherapy, in Comprehensive Textbook of Psychiatry VII. Edited by Kaplan H, Sadock B. Baltimore, MD, Williams & Wilkins, 1999, pp 2225–2234

Gabbard GO: Psychodynamic Psychiatry in Clinical Practice, 3rd Edition. Washington, DC, American Psychiatric Press, 2000

Gabbard GO: Psychoanalysis and psychoanalytic psychotherapy, in Handbook of Personality Disorders. Edited by Livesley J. New York, Guilford (in press)

Gabbard GO, Bartlett AB: Selective serotonin reuptake inhibitors in the context of an ongoing analysis. Psychoanalytic Inquiry 18:657–672, 1998

Gabbard GO, Wilkinson SM: Management of Countertransference With Borderline Patients. Washington, DC, American Psychiatric Press, 1994

Goldberg RS, Reba M, Tasman A: Psychiatrists' attitudes toward prescribing medication for patients treated by nonmedical psychotherapists. Hospital and Community Psychiatry 42:276–280, 1991

Goldberg SE, Schulz S, Schulz PM, et al: Borderline and schizotypal personality disorders treated with low-dose thiothixene vs placebo. Arch Gen Psychiatry 43:680–686, 1986

Gunderson JG, Links P: Borderline personality disorder, in Treatments of Psychiatric Disorders, 2nd Edition. Edited by Gabbard GO. Washington, DC, American Psychiatric Press, 1995, pp 2291–2309

Gunderson JG, Phillips KA: A current view of the interface between borderline personality disorder and depression. Am J Psychiatry 148:967–975, 1991

Gunderson JG, Frank AF, Ronningstam EF, et al: Early discontinuance of borderline patients from psychotherapy. J Nerv Ment Dis 177:38–42, 1989

Gunderson JG, Triebwaser JT, Phillips KA, et al: Personality and vulnerability to affective disorders, in Personality and Psychopathology. Edited by Cloninger CR. Washington, DC, American Psychiatric Press, 1999, pp 3–32

Hollander E: Managing aggressive behavior in patients with obsessive-compulsive disorder and borderline personality disorder. Journal of Clinical Psychiatry Monograph 17:28–31, 1999

Jonas JM, Pope HG: Axis I comorbidity of borderline personality disorder: clinical implications, in Borderline Personality Disorder: Clinical and Empirical Perspectives. Edited by Clarkin JF, Marziali E, Munroe-Blum H. New York, Guilford, 1992, pp 149–160

Kapfhammer H-P, Hippius H: Special feature: pharmacotherapy in personality disorders. J Personal Disord 12:277–288, 1998

Koenigsberg HW: The role of medication in the treatment of borderline personality disorder, in Supportive Therapy for Borderline Patients: A Psychodynamic Approach. Edited by Rockland LH. New York, Guilford, 1992, pp 254–268

Koenigsberg HW: The combination of psychotherapy and pharmacotherapy in the treatment of borderline patients. Journal of Psychotherapy Practice and Research 3:93–107, 1994

Liebowitz MR, Quitkin FM, Stewart JW, et al: Antidepressant specificity in atypical depression. Arch Gen Psychiatry 45:129–137, 1988

Liebowitz MR, Schneier FR, Campeas R, et al: Phenelzine vs atenolol in social phobia: a placebo controlled comparison. Arch Gen Psychiatry 49:290–300, 1992

Linehan MM, Armstrong HE, Suarez A, et al: Cognitive-behavioral treatment of chronically parasuicidal borderline patients. Arch Gen Psychiatry 48:1060–1064, 1991

Links PS, Steiner M, Boiago I, et al: Lithium therapy for borderline patients: preliminary findings. J Personal Disord 4:173–181, 1990

Links PS, Heslegrave R, Villella J: Psychopharmacological management of personality disorders: an outcome-focused model, in Biology of Personality Disorders (Review of Psychiatry Series, Vol 17; Oldham JM, Riba MB, series eds). Edited by Silk KR. Washington, DC, American Psychiatric Press, 1998, pp 93–127

Marcus ER: Integrating psychopharmacotherapy, psychotherapy, and mental structure in the treatment of patients with personality disorders and depression. Psychiatr Clin North Am 13:255–263, 1990

Markovitz PJ: Pharmacotherapy of impulsivity, aggression, and related disorders, in Impulsivity and Aggression. Edited by Hollander E, Stein DJ. New York, Wiley, 1995, pp 263–287

Meares R, Stevenson J, Comerford A: Psychotherapy with borderline patients, I: a comparison between treated and untreated cohorts. Aust N Z J Psychiatry 33:467–472, 1999

Meyer DJ, Simon RI: Split treatment: clarity between psychiatrists and psychotherapists, part I. Psychiatric Annals 29:241–245, 1999a

Meyer DJ, Simon RI: Split treatment: clarity between psychiatrists and psychotherapists, part II. Psychiatric Annals 29:327–332, 1999b

Pfohl B, Stangl D, Zimmerman M: The implications of DSM-III personality disorders for patients with major depression. J Affect Disord 7:309–318, 1984

Rogers JH, Widiger TA, Krupp A: Aspects of depression associated with borderline personality disorder. Am J Psychiatry 152:268–270, 1995

Roth AS, Ostroff RB, Hoffman RE: Naltrexone as a treatment for repetitive self-injurious behavior: an open-label trial. J Clin Psychiatry 57:233–237, 1996

Salzman C, Wolfson AN, Schatzberg A, et al: Effect of fluoxetine on anger in symptomatic volunteers with borderline personality disorder. J Clin Psychopharmacol 15:23–29, 1995

Sederer LI, Ellison J, Keyes C: Guidelines for prescribing psychiatrists in consultative, collaborative, and supervisory relationships. Psychiatr Serv 49:1197–1202, 1998

Serban G, Siegel S: Response of borderline and schizotypal patients to small doses of thiothixene and haloperidol. Am J Psychiatry 141:1455–1458, 1984

Shea MT, Widiger TA, Klein MH: Comorbidity of personality disorders and depression: implications for treatment. J Consult Clin Psychol 60:857–868, 1992

Siever LS, Davis KL: A psychobiologic perspective on the personality disorders. Am J Psychiatry 148:1647–1658, 1991

Soloff PH: Algorithms for pharmacological treatment of personality dimensions: symptom-specific treatments for cognitive-perceptual, affective, and impulsive-behavioral dysregulation. Bull Menninger Clin 62:195–214, 1998

Soloff PH, George A, Nathan RS, et al: Progress in pharmacotherapy of borderline disorders: a double-blind study of amitriptyline, haloperidol, and placebo. Arch Gen Psychiatry 43:691–697, 1986

Soloff PH, George A, Nathan RS, et al: Amitriptyline versus haloperidol in borderlines: final outcomes and predictors of response. J Clin Psychopharmacol 9:238–246, 1989

Soloff PH, Cornelius J, George A, et al: Efficacy of phenelzine and haloperidol in borderline personality disorder. Arch Gen Psychiatry 50:377–395, 1993

Stein MB, Liebowitz MR, Lydiard RB, et al: Paroxetine treatment of generalized social phobia (social anxiety disorder): a randomized controlled trial. JAMA 280:708–713, 1998

Stevenson J, Meares R: An outcome study of psychotherapy for patients with borderline personality disorder. Am J Psychiatry 149:358–362, 1992

Stone MH: The Fate of Borderline Patients: Successful Outcome and Psychiatric Practice. New York, Guilford, 1990

Svrakic DM, Whitehead C, Pryzbeck TR, et al: Differential diagnosis of personality disorders by the seven-factor model of temperament and character. Arch Gen Psychiatry 50:991–999, 1993

Tyrer P, Gunderson J, Lyons M, et al: Extent of comorbidity between mental state and personality disorders. J Personal Disord 11:242–259, 1997

Versiani M, Nardi AE, Mundim FD, et al: Pharmacotherapy of social phobia: a controlled study with moclobemide and phenelzine. Br J Psychiatry 161:353–360, 1992

Waldinger RJ, Frank AF: Transference and the vicissitudes of medication use by borderline patients. Psychiatry 52:416–427, 1989

Winston A, Laikin M, Pollack J, et al: Short-term psychotherapy of personality disorders. Am J Psychiatry 151:190–194, 1994

Woodward B, Duckworth KS, Gutheil TG: The pharmacotherapist-psychotherapist collaboration, in American Psychiatric Press Review of Psychiatry, Vol 12. Edited by Oldham JM, Riba MB, Tasman A. Washington, DC, American Psychiatric Press, 1993, pp 631–649

Woody GE, McLellan T, Luborsky L, et al: Sociopathy and psychotherapy outcome. Arch Gen Psychiatry 42:1081–1086, 1985

Zimmerman M, Coryell W: DSM-III personality disorder diagnoses in a nonpatient sample: demographic correlates and comorbidity. Arch Gen Psychiatry 46:682–689, 1989

Chapter 4

Gradations of Antisociality and Responsivity to Psychosocial Therapies

Michael H. Stone, M.D.

Antisocial personality disorder is a serious condition affecting some 1.5% of the American population. The sex ratio is staggered disproportionately toward the male side (male-to-female ratio of at least 2:1; some estimates cite a ratio of as high as 8:1). Any condition discernible in 3–4 million Americans cannot be uniform in its clinical presentation. The DSM-IV (American Psychiatric Association 1994) definition is itself polythetic, meaning that many combinations of seven defining traits and behaviors (at least three must be present) converge to yield the diagnosis (see Table 4–1). The diagnosis ranges from a fairly mild and correctable disorder to a lethal, incurable one. The combination "2-3-6" (deceitful/impulsive/irresponsible), for example, poses less threat of physical harm; persons manifesting "4-5-7" are prone to assaultiveness.

Some antisocial acts are carried out by persons who were behaving uncharacteristically or impulsively yet not within the context of a confirmed antisocial personality disorder per se. A whole spectrum of behavior patterns is possible. This spectrum begins in the general population at one end, for which no special treatment methods are even indicated, and ends at the most severe and menacing problems, for which no treatment methods are even effective. Clinicians need to know where, along this spectrum, the cutoff band between treatability and nontreatability is. Researchers need to know how to better evaluate antisocial persons, so as to predict with ever greater accuracy 1) who may be amenable to

Table 4–1. DSM-IV diagnostic criteria for antisocial personality disorder

A. There is a pervasive pattern of disregard for and violation of the rights of others occurring since age 15 years, as indicated by three (or more) of the following:
  (1) failure to conform to social norms with respect to lawful behaviors as indicated by repeatedly performing acts that are grounds for arrest
  (2) deceitfulness, as indicated by repeated lying, use of aliases, or conning others for personal profit or pleasure
  (3) impulsivity or failure to plan ahead
  (4) irritability and aggressiveness, as indicated by repeated physical fights or assaults
  (5) reckless disregard for safety of self or others
  (6) consistent irresponsibility, as indicated by repeated failure to sustain consistent work behavior or honor financial obligations
  (7) lack of remorse, as indicated by being indifferent to or rationalizing having hurt, mistreated, or stolen from another
B. The individual is at least age 18 years.
C. There is evidence of conduct disorder with onset before age 15 years.
D. The occurrence of antisocial behavior is not exclusively during the course of schizophrenia or a manic episode.

Source. Reprinted from American Psychiatric Association: *Diagnostic and Statistical Manual of Mental Disorders,* Fourth Edition. Washington, DC, American Psychiatric Association, 1994. Used with permission. Copyright © 1994 American Psychiatric Association.

treatment, 2) who will probably drop their antisocial behaviors with time (albeit remaining unresponsive to therapy beforehand), and 3) who will likely remain on the far side of treatability altogether.

Treatment resources will always be scarce, compared with the large number of chronic offenders (and the even larger number of mildly antisocial persons who manage not to get into serious trouble with the law). It is both sound fiscal policy and ethically defensible that we mobilize our therapeutic resources primarily on behalf of those with a better likelihood of response, so as not

Table 4–2. Gradations of antisociality

1. Some antisocial personality traits that are insufficient to meet DSM criteria; some antisocial traits occurring in another personality disorder
2. Explosive irritable personality disorder with some antisocial traits
3. Malignant narcissism
4. Antisocial personality disorder with property crimes only
5. Sexual offenses without violence (i.e., voyeurism, exhibitionism, frotteurism)
6. Antisocial personality disorder with violent felonies (some psychopathic traits may be present but are insufficient to meet Hare's Psychopathy Checklist—Revised criteria: score > 29)
7. Psychopathy without violence (e.g., con artists, financial scams)
8. Psychopathy with violent crimes
9. Psychopathy with sadistic control (e.g., unlawful imprisonment of a kidnap victim while awaiting ransom)
10. Psychopathy with violent sadism and murder but no prolonged torture
11. Psychopathy with prolonged torture followed by murder

to impair their chances for rehabilitation by having devoted our resources to those least likely to become responsible citizens.

To this end, I have envisioned a series of antisocial behavior patterns, which can be well ordered into a schema that I refer to as the *gradations of antisociality* (Table 4–2).

At the mildest end of this spectrum are persons, usually in their younger years, who engage in school truancy, steal small amounts of money, shoplift, or commit minor acts of vandalism. Such behaviors may be infrequent and may occur within the context of another personality disorder or specifiable condition or perhaps in the absence of any diagnosis in DSM's latest edition. Strictly speaking, antisocial personality disorder is not to be diagnosed, according to DSM-IV, before age 18 years, although some attributes of conduct disorder may have been present before age 15 years. Among the four categories of conduct disorder outlined in DSM-IV (aggression to people and animals, destruction of property, deceitfulness or theft, and serious violations of rules), minor acts of theft or property destruction may be the easiest to remedy; patterns of aggressivity may be the most difficult (and certainly the most serious). The school bully at age 8 years, for example, often will be arrested for an offense by age 28 (Huesman et al. 1984).

The path from severe conduct disorder in latency and adolescence to antisocial personality disorder after age 18 is commonly seamless and uninterrupted. Among adults who fulfill criteria for a personality disorder, those most likely to show some antisocial traits (apart from persons with antisocial personality disorder proper) are those with the other Cluster B disorders: borderline, narcissistic, or histrionic. A degree of overlap also exists between paranoid personality disorder and antisocial personality disorder (or some of its traits). Examples of the latter would be paranoid fanatics who engage in acts of bigotry and destruction (e.g., letter bombs, poisonings, shootings) against targeted groups.

Gradations of Antisociality

In describing the gradations of what I have called *antisociality* (the tendency to behave in antisocial ways), my guiding variables are amenability to treatment (or to eventual self-correction) and the seriousness of the antisocial tendencies. In this schema, a murderer who was repentant and amenable to therapy would still represent a more serious gradation than an unrepentant shoplifter (as in Vignette 7 below). Assaultive persons who feel genuine remorse eventually may outgrow their assaultive tendencies. This would render their prognosis better than that of certain unscrupulous businessmen who revel in getting away with (fiscal, if not physical) "murder" throughout their life.

Situated between narcissistic personality disorder and antisocial personality disorder, according to the schema of Kernberg (1992) relating to antisociality, is a personality disorder that he designated *malignant narcissism*. Persons with this syndrome show marked narcissistic traits admixed with antisocial behaviors, although not in such variety and pervasiveness as to meet DSM criteria for antisocial personality disorder. These patients also have a paranoid orientation but a simultaneous capacity for loyalty and concern for others.

A critical element within the variable of seriousness is *dangerousness*. With prudence, the average citizen has a good chance of resisting the blandishments of real-estate scam artists, dishonest used-car salespersons, and the like. But even the most cautious may not be immune to the predations of stalkers, rapists, "carjackers," spouse-bashers, or other violent persons who injure, violate, or murder the innocent.

I believe that there is no impressive correlation between the mere number of antisocial personality disorder items and either the prognosis or the level of dangerousness. As for treatability, the methods currently available are not very effective within the entire domain of antisociality. Current methods are effective only at the milder side of the spectrum.

The most dangerous persons are those with strong tendencies toward violence or sadism. However, some persons (predominantly men) with sadistic personality (Stone 1998) and long histories of assaultive behavior meet criteria for antisocial personality disorder but not for *psychopathic* personality (see section "The Concept of Psychopathy" below); others have only a few traits of antisocial personality disorder or psychopathy, and still others have combined sadism, antisocial personality disorder, and psychopathy. In Table 4–2, I used the criterion "Psychopathy with prolonged torture followed by murder" as the extreme band at the severe end of the antisociality spectrum.

Persons with these descriptors are uniformly and predictably dangerous. But admittedly, there are nonpsychopathic persons who, for example, abuse spouses psychologically and physically, molest children sexually, or torment friends and relatives, thus approximating the dangerousness level of the psychopathic torturers, even though they fall short of the extreme band of the spectrum.

Several vignettes below illustrate the various bands along the spectrum. First, the issue of *psychopathy* as distinct from antisocial personality disorder must be addressed.

The Concept of Psychopathy

The term *psychopathy* has undergone significant changes since Kraepelin (1915) sketched several "psychopathic personalities" in his four-volume text. The relevant chapter included persons who were either excitable/irritable, unstable, impulse-ridden, eccentric, liars and cheats, antisocial, or quarrelsome. Etymologically, "psychopathy" merely conveys illness of the mind; the Kraepelinian usage was very broad, and only a portion of his subtypes would be subsumed under the term as it is now used. When Hervey Cleckley (1941) described the "psychopath" in his monograph *The Mask of Sanity*, he confined the term to persons whose chief characteristics were those of superficial charm, untruthfulness, egocentricity, trivialization of their sexual life, lack of remorse, and failure to learn from experience. These psychopaths often engaged in "fantastic and uninviting behavior with drink or sometimes without" (p. 248). Inadequately motivated antisocial behavior was another feature. Such persons were thus self-centered (narcissistic, in contemporary parlance), flamboyant, and contemptuous of social convention and rules. The con artist would be a typical example.

There are important differences between the concepts of antisocial personality disorder and psychopathy. In DSM-III and DSM-III-R (American Psychiatric Association 1980, 1987), antisocial personality disorder was defined mostly via behavioral items, such as truancy, destroying property, and getting into fights. These were not descriptors of personality but rather examples of misbehavior that, although easier to document than subtleties of personality, did not really get to the essence of the antisocial personality. Robert Hare and his colleagues in Canada over the past 20 years have sought to rectify this problem. They revised and amplified the original Cleckley descriptors and performed tests of reliability and validity with the emerging Psychopathy Checklist—Revised (PCL-R) (Hare 1995; Hare et al. 1991; Harpur et al. 1989; Harris et al. 1994; Hart et al. 1994).

The PCL-R consists of 20 items, many of which are true descriptors of personality. These have recently been gathered into a subgroup, answering to the first of two factors into which the checklist can be analyzed. This Factor I consists of intensely narcissistic traits, such as those that impinge uncomfortably on other people, but not the comparatively harmless traits of preoccupation with beauty or wanting to be the center of attention (that form part of the criteria for DSM narcissistic personality disorder).

The Factor I items are

- Glibness; superficial charm
- Grandiose sense of self-worth
- Pathological lying
- Conning/manipulative
- Lack of remorse or guilt
- Shallow affect
- Callous/lack of empathy (what is actually meant here is lack of compassion)
- Failure to accept responsibility for one's actions

In evaluations made with the PCL-R, each item is given a rating of "0," "1," or "2." This yields a maximum score of 40. In the United States and Canada, psychopathy (or psychopathic personality) is diagnosed only if the score is 30 or higher. In parts of Europe, a score of 25 is deemed sufficient.

The concept of psychopathy has several advantages compared with that of antisocial personality as defined in DSM-IV. As af Klinteberg (1998) underlined, psychopathy lends itself to a dimensional approach. As a diagnosis established by the PCL-R, psychopathy has a categorical aspect also, but persons with intermediate scores (in the 7–29 range) may be said to show various degrees (dimensionally speaking) of what he refers to as *psychopathic personality* (p. 140). Psychopathy may usefully be seen, in fact, as a subset largely within the domain of antisocial personality disorder, inasmuch as almost all persons satisfying the Hare criteria for psychopathy also meet those of antisocial personality disorder, whereas only a portion of those with antisocial personality disorder meet the tighter criteria for psychopathy.

Viewing psychopathic personality in dimensional terms makes it easier to understand how, in its mildest forms (in which only a few of the PCL-R items, such as charm, deceitfulness, and grandiosity, are pertinent), the condition blends into the general population, in which many persons with a few such traits function successfully and would not be considered "disordered." M. McGuire and Troisi (1998) make this point in their discussion of antisociality (they do not use the term *psychopathy*) within an *evolutionary* framework. The psychopath in the social context is a "nonreciprocator": someone who deceives and manipulates others to satisfy his or her needs and to get ahead. Successful psychopaths also are adept at eluding detection. This ability to elude detection is enhanced by the psychopath's tendency to migrate from places where he or she becomes too well known to places (including different countries) where he or she is not known (M. McGuire et al. 1994). The psychopath's freedom from guilt permits him or her to act in certain situations in which ordinary persons are inhibited. Likewise, his or her strong need for stimulation (the high novelty-seeking of which Cloninger and colleagues speak [Cloninger 1986; Cloninger et al. 1993] as an attribute of the antisocial personality) and his or her impulsivity (low harm avoidance, in Cloninger's model) make the psychopath a risk-taker. At the milder end of the psychopathic personality continuum, these qualities may contribute to success in the form of superior entrepreneurship in business. Yet at the severe end of this continuum, where we confront the diagnosed psychopath with the high PCL-R score, the condition, far from being adaptive, represents the extreme example of antisociality. This is the territory of the repeat criminal, the stock-fraud swindler, the arsonist for hire, the serial killer, and so on.

Antisocial personality disorder, in contrast, is a broad concept. Not all antisocial persons lack remorse and compassion or are committed to a lifelong course of deceiving others and are therefore less homogeneous with respect to prognosis than are the (PCL-R score 30 or greater) diagnosable psychopaths.

The comparative homogeneity of psychopathy and its adaptive value when present in milder form encourage the search for relevant genetic influences and for biological markers that may reflect such influences. It is important in this regard to note how the forensic group at Ontario's Penetanguishene Mental Health Centre endorse the evolutionary hypothesis of M. McGuire and Troisi (1998), commenting that "Psychopathy may not be a mental disorder at all, but instead an evolved 'cheater' life strategy that contributed to fitness in ancestral environments" by virtue of their "glibness and superficial charm, pathological lying, sexual promiscuity, lack of remorse, shallow affect, impulsivity and irresponsibility" (Harris et al. 1994).

Many studies in recent years have testified to the validity of Hare's definition of psychopathy. Some focused on neurophysiological correlates; others focused on the prediction of offender recidivism. Among the latter is the report of Hemphill et al. (1998), which examined the likelihood that a convicted offender would, on his or her eventual release from prison, still be free in the community and not reconvicted for a new offense within the 12-year span of the study. Released offenders were compartmentalized into three groups, corresponding to low (0–19), medium (20–29), and high (30+) PCL-R scores. By 3 years, only a quarter of the group with high PCL-R scores had not been reconvicted (for *any* type of offense), half of the group with medium PCL-R scores were still free, and three-quarters of the group with low PCL-R scores had not been reconvicted. The same pattern held true for violent recidivism.

Gradations of Antisociality: Clinical and Biographical Vignettes

Vignette 1:
The presence of some nonviolent antisocial traits that are insufficient to meet DSM criteria for antisocial personality disorder, either in the absence or in the presence of another personality disorder

I had occasion to treat in private practice an unmarried 35-year-old woman with borderline personality disorder. She came from a middle-class family and worked as a marketing analyst after graduating from college. She was engaged to a young lawyer whom she sought to control, actually to subjugate completely, via incessant criticisms and by alienating him from all of his friends, who found her abrasiveness intolerable. Inverately hostile and angry toward her parents (who were paying for her therapy), she once returned from visiting them in a towering rage over some trivial matter. She showed me a photograph she had taken of them in which she had gouged out the eyes with an X-acto knife and told me that she was going to send them the altered pictures (against my strong objections) to "get back at them." She did so, and this caused a serious rift with her parents. Next, at a Thanksgiving dinner with her fiancé's family, she proceeded to blurt out: "Tim *has* to marry me, you know, because he gave me genital herpes, and Dr. Stone agrees!" In reality, she had given him herpes, and I of course never sanctioned such blackmail. At that point, I terminated her treatment, and her fiancé finally summoned the courage to break off the engagement.

Vignette 2:
Explosive/irritable personality disorder
with some antisocial traits

A separated electrician had been admitted to a forensic hospital after he had, while in a depressed and agitated state, shot his wife in the buttocks with a rifle. He had helped her financially through law school, where she had met another law student with whom she began an affair. She sued for divorce, moved out, and sought custody of their daughter. When she returned one morning to collect some belongings, he flew into a rage and shot her.

In his early years, his mother, who had reared him alone after his father had abandoned the family, used to berate him cruelly and whip him with an electrical cord for the most minor peccadilloes.

After he shot his wife, he fled to Alabama, where he hid out in a motel for several weeks. While there, he had a "religious experience" in which he heard God's voice telling him to return to New York and to give himself up to the authorities. After doing so, and having been found mentally ill at the time, he was remanded to a forensic hospital. He had no arrest record.

As he grew calmer, he was able to acknowledge that he was hot-tempered and that he occasionally was violent with his wife, in the midst of arguments, as their marriage began to deteriorate. He was fiercely moralistic and, in fact, was fanatic about the unbreakable nature of the marital bond (even when the two parties could not get along), and he regarded his wife as sinful for seeking divorce. He claimed that he had no intention of killing her and merely wanted to wound her (which he did), although he admitted that his mind often was filled with murderous fantasies prompted by her infidelity. The only patient on my unit to express genuine remorse for what he had done, and to grasp the connection between the past (his hatred of his mother) and the present (taking this hatred out on his wife), he rapidly reintegrated and was returned to the court for trial.

Vignette 3:
Malignant narcissism

A 45-year-old married man sought treatment because of his rage outbursts both at work and at home with his wife. In addition to his explosive, irritable personality, he was grandiose, was a tyrannical boss of the company he had founded, and humiliated his employees, reducing them to tears, for minor shortcomings. At home, if his wife criticized such behavior or prepared supper late, he would suddenly sweep all the crockery off the table or kick down the doors in their apartment. Similar outbursts occurred at work, such that many employees, terrified, quit their jobs.

He had many bipolar traits and had come from a family with several bipolar members. In his better moments, he could be effusive with praise, witty, charming, and seductive; in fact, he was a "Don Juan," with many brief affairs in various countries. He had been married twice before. His mood gyrated between murderously hostile (vowing with great determination that he would kill "that bitch of a wife") and tearfully dependent ("I'm nothing without her"). He felt genuine hatred toward both his family and his in-laws, yet he was loyal to his friends and to the few employees who managed to work up to his demanding standards. On the occasions when he struck his wife, he felt intense guilt shortly afterward. He was willing to take mood stabilizers and antidepressants, which in time curbed, but did not eliminate, his aggressive tendencies.

Vignette 4:
Antisocial personality disorder with property crimes only

The husband of a patient I had been treating had been fired from his post as an investment banker in a large firm. Smug, deceitful, psychologically unreflective, and much less capable than he pictured himself, he had overstayed a vacation for many days without notifying the firm. This had been the "last straw" for his superiors. It then became apparent that he had been having an affair with a younger friend of his wife. She sued for divorce at this point; he pled poverty, as though unable to make child support payments, despite his showering his new inamorata with expensive baubles.

My patient had this paradox investigated. It turned out that he had recently been named executor for the estate of a millionairess who had just died. He managed to wrangle power of attorney from the estate and then began siphoning off large sums of money, well in excess of the executor's fee to which he was legally entitled. Again pleading poverty, he demanded half the value of their house, even though it was in his wife's name, on the grounds that she was employed and he was not, and she "owed" him half the value on the grounds of "communal marital property." He lost the case but tied up her assets for many months and caused her to lose considerable sums for her legal defense. He did not pay a penny in child support but nevertheless demanded to see the children regularly, even though when they came to his place, he spent no time with them, making the elder child (then 12) baby-sit for the younger children while he and his now fiancée stepped out for the evening.

Vignette 5:
Sexual offenses without violence

In a case reported by Wayne Myers (1991), a married man sought treatment for marital problems, complicated by two forms of sexual perversion: making obscene telephone calls and practicing frotteurism to orgasm while traveling in the subway. He was born with blindness in one eye and a spinal deformity and had always felt that these were signs of "unmanliness." He had grown up in a large family with many siblings, and he complained that his mother had seemed indifferent to him.

Both he and his wife were "problem drinkers": it was usually when he had been drinking, and when he had been angry at his wife, that he would go into the subway and rub himself against the backside of a female passenger until he achieved orgasm. At other times, under similar circumstances, he would make obscene telephone calls or breathe in a panting, sexual way into the telephone without saying anything.

Myers conducted a largely psychoanalytically oriented therapy for 3 years, during which time the sexual symptomatic behavior diminished. In the meantime, the treatment had focused on his inordinate anger at women in general, beginning with his mother and coming to include his wife and "stranger women" who were the symbolic equivalents of mother and wife and against whom he had felt safer to vent his hostility. Although he was unusually meek and passive apart from when he had been drinking, he had occasionally struck his wife when his anger at her was particularly intense. In other respects, he was a highly regarded middle executive in a large company. He felt considerable guilt over his aggressiveness toward his wife and over the sexual perversions. This guilt provided motivation for his therapy, and by the third year, he no longer drank and no longer practiced either perversion. His relationship with his wife also had improved.

Vignette 6:
Antisocial personality disorder with violent felonies

A 55-year-old married man with two children had been born into a well-to-do home that was characterized by severe marital strife, with constant arguments between his parents. His mother was abrasive and nagging, and his father was ineffectual and permissive but went to great lengths to "preserve peace" or to bail his son, Bernard, out of trouble. Trouble began in Bernard's adolescence, when he began to bully younger students at his school. This led to confrontations with his parents by the school authorities, but no action was taken. He flunked out of his first year of college and took a job in merchandising. This was the first of many brief jobs because his personality—contemptuous and brusque—caused him to be fired from one firm after another. He racked up huge credit card debts, some of which were to raise cash for playing the horses. After being arrested on several occasions for nonpayment, he appealed to his father, who paid sometimes $30,000 or $50,000 to avoid letting Bernard go to prison. The pattern persisted, however, and Bernard then borrowed large sums from Mafia sources but was unable to repay the huge vigorish (usurious interest rates), falling afoul of men who threatened bodily harm. His father again came to the rescue.

Bernard then married a woman he barely knew and moved to a different state. He lied to her about his income, professed to have money in secret accounts, and lived well beyond his means. She finally sued for divorce after 10 years of marriage. He grew enraged at her for leaving him, and one day when she returned to his apartment to have him sign some papers, he shot her to death in front of their daughter.

He had been in treatment in his 20s to no avail.

He was arrested quickly after the murder and insisted on being his own lawyer but so offended the jury that they convicted him of murder one and recommended the death penalty.

Vignette 7:
Psychopathy without violence

Ms. C, a 48-year-old woman, sought to regain custody of her 8-year-old daughter, who was now living with her father (Ms. C's fifth ex-husband) and his new wife. Ms. C had gotten through life since adolescence on her looks and seductiveness and had already had five abortions by as many men by the time she was 20. She never attended college, although she told people she had graduated in "hotel administration" from a prestigious university. The men who became her husbands were led to believe she was wealthy, but each relationship began with a request for $30,000 or $40,000 "to tide her over till the interest on her bonds came into her bank." Each soon found himself caught up in a torrid sexual affair, and by the time it became apparent that she had no such funds, an engagement ring was already on her finger, and the debt was forgiven.

Ms. C was a chronic alcoholic and cocaine user; she was arrested many times for dealing drugs and for driving while intoxicated, but she got the charges dropped by seducing the prosecuting attorney or some other influential politico in her hometown.

Her fourth husband divorced her after she told him she was "pregnant" and that he had to marry her; he had had a vasectomy, unbeknownst to her. Unbeknownst to him, she had not been pregnant anyway. Her fifth husband divorced her after she began blackmailing him. He was granted custody of their daughter and moved to a different state. Ms. C would send her daughter huge packages of toys and clothes, all shoplifted with the tags still on them. When her daughter would visit her for a week or two, Ms. C would take the girl "shopping" and would steal clothes in front of her. She once persuaded her son by her second marriage to dress in her clothes and drive her car, so that when the police tried to collar her for a driving while intoxicated offense, they found that the driver was not Ms. C at all but her son. She had no remorse for her actions.

Vignette 8:
Psychopathy with violent crimes

Sante Kimes, as mentioned by her biographer Adrian Havill (1999), was born Sante Louise Singh in 1934. Her father was a sharecropper in Oklahoma, originally from the Calcutta region; her mother was Irish. After her father abandoned the family when she was 3 years old, her mother became a prostitute. At age 13, she was adopted by a Colonel Chambers. She had already been sexually abused at age 8 years and arrested for stealing at 9 years. For a time, she was law-abiding while with the Chamberses but soon began shoplifting and using their credit cards illegally. She married and divorced several times, each briefly, by age 22. She told people she had graduated from college but had actually never attended.

She was arrested many times in her 20s for theft and used a bewildering array of aliases. Eventually, she used her charms and beauty to seduce a married multimillionaire, by whom she had an illegitimate son, Keith, named after his father, Kenneth Keith Kimes. Later, she assumed the Kimes last name herself. Although she lived in great style while supported by Kimes, she stole "for the thrill of it." When her son was old enough, she used him as an accomplice; in 1980, at a fancy party in Washington, DC, she stole a $10,000 mink coat by wearing it under her own coat and then slipping it to her son. She evaded trial for the theft until 1985 and then skipped town when the guilty verdict was read. She and Kenneth became notorious as "grifters," preying on the gullible wealthy. They stole from a banker in the Cayman Islands, who "disappeared"—presumably killed by them. Recently, Kenneth ingratiated himself into the good graces of a millionaire widow, Irene Silverman, in New York City. The 82-year-old woman also disappeared. Evidence pointing to her murder by the pair was found, and they were finally captured after a long search. They are now facing trial for the widow's murder.

Vignette 9:
Psychopathy with sadistic control

Cameron Hooker, whose history was sketched by C. McGuire and Norton (1988), was born in 1953 to an unremarkable working class family in rural northeast California. The elder of two brothers, Cameron had never been abused or beaten and had always been well cared for. His parents were hard-working religious people with a solid marriage. Gawky and unsure of his looks as an adolescent, Cameron began to elaborate strong fantasies of a sadomasochistic nature in which he assumed total control over women, on whom he forced sex while they were bound up or suspended from the limbs of a tree. He became obsessed with sadomasochistic pornography.

At age 19, he seduced a much younger girl, Janice, whom he later married but not before inducing this very dependent girl to endure being tied up, tied to the ground, hung from a tree by her wrists, and at times beaten (although only hard enough to make welts) with a whip. His sadism intensified after their marriage: he would choke her to unconsciousness or put a knife to her throat. Finally, he decided he needed a third person to complete the living out of his fantasies. To this end, he kidnapped a 20-year-old hitchhiker, Coleen Stan. At first, he kept her tied up in the basement. Then he constructed a large coffinlike box in which he imprisoned her and used her for sex when he so chose. He kept the box under the marital bed; at the beginning, he let Coleen out for brief periods to do various tasks as a slave of the household. Toward the end of her 7-year imprisonment, he kept her in the box almost all the time so that she would not be detected by his two children or by neighbors. Janice and Coleen eventually escaped and were rescued by the police. Cameron was arrested, convicted, and sentenced to 104 years in prison. He is one of the few violent and sadistic psychopaths without a history of childhood maltreatment and was considered an unexplained genetic oddity, a "bad seed" child.

Vignette 10:
Psychopathy with violent sadism and
murder but no prolonged torture

Ted Bundy, one of the most notorious serial killers of the modern era, was born in 1946 in Philadelphia, Pennsylvania. He was an illegitimate child of a woman from a respectable family, but mystery about the circumstances continues, and he may have been the product of incest via his violent grandfather (Michaud and Aynesworth 1983).

His mother moved with her son to Seattle, Washington, and married a cook. Bundy did fairly well academically but since early childhood was oversensitive, self-conscious, and preoccupied with fantasies of wealth and fame. He felt ashamed of his stepfather's working-class status and even more ashamed about his illegitimacy. Neither parent abused or mistreated him.

He got in trouble for lying and stealing at an early age. In his late teens, he fell in love with a beautiful girl from a wealthy family. Although she accepted to become his fiancée, after a time she grew tired of his immaturity and rejected him. This sent him on a downward spiral. He began to steal and shoplift more aggressively and became addicted to violent pornography and voyeurism, especially after he saw a girl undressing in a lighted room. In the meantime, he graduated from college with an undistinguished record, and after several failures was accepted at a law school.

He had a charming facade and a glib tongue. By the early 1970s, he began to stalk women and force his way into their apartments. His first sexual homicide was in 1974, after breaking into a student dormitory and clubbing a young woman to death. Bundy became a master at deception, luring women into his car by wearing one arm in a sling and asking for help with large packages when coming from a shopping mall. Once the woman helped Bundy and got in the car to deposit the package, her fate was sealed. The passenger door locked, and he drove the woman off to a secluded area, where he raped and killed his victim and then hid the body. Over the next 4 years, before his capture, he killed at least 19 women.

Vignette 11:
*Psychopathy with prolonged
torture followed by murder*

Herman Mudgett, alias Henry H. Holmes, was born in 1860 to a prosperous New Hampshire farm family of devout Methodist background. He had two brothers who led normal lives, and no history of abusive upbringing was found (Franke 1975). He went to medical school, before and after which he had several unsuccessful businesses.

He relocated to Chicago, Illinois, and began constructing a 90-room "castle," with ordinary shops on the ground floor, but built in such a way as to contain trapdoors, rooms without exits, blind hallways, secret passages, and lime pits in the cellar. A consummate con man, lady-charmer, bigamist, and insurance swindler, he lured unsuspecting secretaries and other women to work for him. He then quickly persuaded them to marry him but not before they exchanged insurance policies on which each became the beneficiary of the other "if anything should happen." He would then overpower them after a night of lovemaking and propel them through a trapdoor into a torture chamber. After his fantasies were sated, he would kill the women and dump their bodies into the lime pit to disappear gradually. The number of his victims has never been determined accurately and ranges from about 30 to 200, depending on which account one reads.

Mudgett/Holmes had maintained three wives in as many cities, each thinking his absences (to see one of the others) were for a business trip. He was handsome, charming, and apparently idolized by each wife as a wonderful, if too often absent, husband.

He was apprehended in 1895 and was hanged a year later. A paradigm case of psychopathy, Mudgett's criminal record has scarcely been surpassed in the century that has followed. Given the innocuousness of his upbringing, one can only conclude that he represents a genetic anomaly, someone born with the extremes of brain factors that predispose to novelty-seeking, lack of compassion, and a taste for violence.

Gradations of Antisociality: Implications for Treatment

Any discussion of treatment within the domain of antisociality is necessarily complicated by multiple factors, such as the age of the potential patient, the underlying character structure, the degree of motivation (often sorely lacking in antisocial persons), the chronicity of the antisocial behavior patterns, the seriousness of the offenses committed (especially in cases of sexual offenses, in which repetitive offenses are the rule), and as a corollary to the latter, the gravity of problems with the law, the strength of any propensity to violence, the nature of any arrest record, the variety of criminal acts engaged in, and the degree to which psychopathic traits dominate the personality profile. Cultural factors also figure in the equation. In certain subcultures and social groups, adherence to a code of honor and loyalty is strictly adhered to *within* the group, but outsiders are considered "fair game" for predation. The members of such groups are often "normal" viewed within the context of the other members yet share with psychopaths the conviction that they themselves are perfectly fine and in no need of help from the psychiatric profession. They thus lack "caseness," epidemiologically speaking, and would certainly not count themselves as examples of persons with personality disorder.

Table 4–2 proceeds generally from the prognostically more hopeful to the least hopeful subtypes. But even here it is not easy to construct a straightforward continuum, except when one has crossed over into the region of psychopathy. There, not only amenability to treatment is negligible or nonexistent but also the tendency to "burn out" when past age 40—as one sees with nonpsychopathic antisocial personality disorder (Robins et al. 1991)—is scarcely in evidence.

The lack of caseness that applies to the members of certain subcultures is also a factor in the much larger group of persons who violate the trust of, and inflict serious psychological or physical harm to, their children. Almost 2 million child abuse victims are known in the United States, and presumably a comparable number of parents or caregivers are responsible for this maltreatment. But only the most egregious examples are ever brought before justice. The remainder—perpetrators of incest, child beating, sadistic humiliation, and the like—go either undetected, unpunished, or untreated. Some examples are truly horrific, as in the case of Mary Bell in England's Newcastle upon Tyne.

At age 11, Mary Bell murdered two small boys and was then demonized, according to her biographer, Gitta Sereny (1998), as the "incarnation of evil," as "bad seed" personified. But Mary Bell, who was eventually rehabilitated, and now lives an exemplary life (under an assumed name) with a daughter of her own, was no "bad seed." The family member with the psychopathic traits was not the youthful murderess but rather her prostitute mother, who tried to kill Mary on many occasions during the first years of her life. When Mary was 5 or 6 years old, her mother forced her to perform fellatio on the mother's "clients," to submit to having objects forced into her rectum, and to endure whippings. Betty, her mother, warned Mary of dire consequences if she ever told anyone. A few years later, Betty tried to drown her daughter and also throttled her into unconsciousness on several occasions. It was these assaults that were reenacted when Mary strangled the two boys. The point here is that Betty was never brought to justice and never treated (assuming a treatment for such aberrations of personality exist) for the crimes against her daughter. Thus, it is no surprise that Mary Bell behaved in a highly aggressive manner during her early years, becoming a "made" rather than a "born" antisocial person.

Lack of caseness is also a factor in certain instances of antisocial, or even psychopathic, offspring in families of great wealth or social prominence. Criminal activities by young persons from such families sometimes are papered over, the investigating authorities are intimidated or bought off, or the family successfully stonewalls the police behind a barricade of attorneys. The value of any goods stolen can quickly be compensated by cash payments to the victims, so that no lawsuit ever occurs. Murder and rape can go unprosecuted, or the sentence rendered nugatory, as in the case of Jennifer Levin's murderer, Robert Chambers (Taubman 1988). As a result, ratings of the offenders in these circumstances may be artificially lowered to levels beneath the "radar" of the PCL-R, yielding a false-negative (<30) reading.

Treatment for the Treatable

What qualities in persons with severe conduct disorders in early life, with established antisocial personality disorder later on, or with subclinical forms of antisocial personality disorder such as malignant narcissism or just a few antisocial traits make a favorable outcome (with or without treatment) possible? The best answer we can offer at present, I believe, is found not so much in this or that diagnostic *category* but in the *absence* of certain Factor I psychopathic traits. Glibness and superficial charm, or grandiosity, do not augur well for a good therapeutic alliance (in any form of therapy) but do not, in the absence of the other Factor I traits, spell the defeat of our therapeutic efforts.

Treatability in the domain of antisociality depends, it would appear, on the presence of adequate motivation and on the ability to take seriously the nature of one's antisocial attitudes and behaviors.

Treatability also requires the *absence* of 1) pathological lying/deceitfulness, 2) conning/manipulativeness, 3) lack of remorse or guilt, and 4) callousness/lack of compassion. These four traits represent the core of the special and extreme form of narcissism—*predatory* narcissism, as distinct from the mere vanity of the nonpredatory narcissist—that constitutes the essence of psychopathy. Related to the lack of remorse trait is contemptuousness: the disregard for the feelings of others, coupled with the devaluation of other persons. That includes of course the devaluation of potential treaters within the mental health profession, whom the psychopath looks on as "suckers," "fools," or "wimps."

From Sereny's biography, it is clear that Mary Bell, despite the animal torture and the double murders in her 11th year, possessed a core of compassion and of decency of character, with the absence of the predatory narcissistic traits enumerated above. This constellation of personality allowed her, thanks also to the warmth and wisdom of her caregivers in the reformatory she was sent to after her trial, to make a good social recovery. Even someone who has committed murder will be easier to treat, given those favorable traits, than a psychopath with strong Factor I traits who has never been violent. Statistically, to be sure, psychopathic offenders are three to four times as likely to be violent than are nonpsychopathic offenders (Hare and McPherson 1984).

Another set of guidelines concerning treatability, cast in the negative, stems from the work of the forensic psychologist J. Reid Meloy (1988). He offered five contraindications to psychotherapy for violent patients: 1) a history of sadistic behavior with injury, 2) a complete absence of remorse, 3) an IQ indicating either superior intelligence or retarded, 4) a lack of capacity for attachment (similar to schizoid aloofness), and 5) an intense countertransference fear of predation in the therapist (i.e., of being stalked, threatened, or injured).

As for ideal qualities in the therapist working with antisocial patients, Gabbard (1994) offered six recommendations. The therapist must 1) be incorruptible, stable, and persistent; 2) confront repeatedly the patient's denial and minimization of his or her antisocial behavior; 3) help the patient connect his or her actions with his or her internal (emotional/attitudinal) states; 4) confront the here-and-now behaviors (as more effective than interpretations about the past); 5) monitor countertransference so as to avoid inappropriate responses; and 6) avoid excessive expectations for improvement. Gabbard's remarks are an excellent summary of the ideal qualities in shaping dynamic psychotherapy for antisocial patients, although they also hold true for therapists relying on other approaches.

In general, a dynamic therapy, even focusing on the here and now, is useful only for a minority of persons with antisocial personality disorder: those with some remnants of genuine concern for others and of remorse about their actions. A greater number of borderline patients who have a few antisocial features (shoplifting, reckless driving, substance abuse with some minor dealing), short of full antisocial personality disorder comorbidity, also will be amenable to dynamic psychotherapy, provided habitual lying is *not* one of those antisocial traits. The chronically deceitful patient has, after all, surrounded himself or herself with an impenetrable camouflage, behind which the "real" person is undiscoverable.

The malignant narcissist also may become a workable patient with dynamic therapy (including the transference-focused psychotherapy developed by Clarkin and colleagues [1999]), provided the patient has not garnered for himself or herself the invincible armor of political or financial power, which radically diminishes any feeling of a need for psychiatric help.

These guidelines also apply to work with forensic patients, in whom the character structure underlying a psychosis is the key factor determining treatability. Two contrasting examples follow:

> A young man with an acute bipolar psychosis developed the delusion that his father was the "Devil" and must be destroyed. He bought a machete and beheaded his household pets and then his father.

In actuality, his father had brutalized both the patient and the patient's brother. The patient's underlying character was that of a wholesome person with a capacity for attachment to others and for genuine remorse about what he had done. After a few years in the forensic hospital while receiving a regimen of lithium, he recovered and was released to a conventional psychiatric facility to continue his rehabilitation.

> A schizophrenic man who had stabbed his girlfriend to death in a fit of jealousy developed the delusion that the Mafia had implanted pieces of metal in his brain in order to monitor his movements.

Twelve years later, in the forensic hospital where he receives a maximum regimen of neuroleptics, he continues to harbor the same delusion and argues that the woman deserved to die because she was "cheating" on him. He is without remorse and is still considered a dangerously mentally ill person.

Cognitive Therapy With Antisocial Persons

Beck and Freeman (1990) discussed antisocial personality disorder from the standpoint of cognitive development, pointing out how antisocial persons appear frozen at a very early stage of Kohlberg's hierarchy of moral maturation (Kohlberg 1984). Such persons inhabit a realm similar to that of latency-age children: "they cannot hold another's point of view at the same time as their own. As such, they cannot take on the role of another" (Beck and Freeman 1990, p. 151). This deficit is reflected in the PCL-R as "lack of empathy." The authors then describe some of the common cognitive distortions typical of persons with antisocial personality disorder—distortions that cognitive therapy will consequently attempt to correct. They enumerate six examples: 1) feeling justified in getting whatever one wants (or in dodging whatever one does not want), 2) thinking is believing (i.e., having an unwavering belief in the accuracy of one's thoughts), 3) personal infallibility, 4) unquestioning acceptance of one's feelings as providing a correct basis for action, 5) view of others as impotent or worthless (their opinions or objections are irrelevant), and 6) minimization of possible untoward consequences.

Although Beck and Freeman mention Hare's checklist and use the term *psychopath,* the cognitive approach they advocate has no relevance to the true psychopath (if defined by a PCL-R score of 30 or higher). Their method is appropriate for patients with antisocial personality disorder who still retain some of the above-mentioned character attributes that permit therapy to go forward. The authors use a method based on the (correct) assumption that antisocial persons are quite capable of making risk-benefit evaluations of various life situations. Ordinarily, they make poor choices because of a hurried and inadequate assessment of the long-term consequences. They live and operate in an endless present. Beck and Freeman give some examples of how a therapist might help a workable antisocial patient improve his or her risk-benefit assessments; they concede that there is nevertheless little likelihood that the patient would ever truly internalize a higher moral value system, one in which the better choices would be made without external coaxing. In one example,

> A patient was placed on probation at work, presumably because of lateness or poor performance. The cognitive therapist encourages the man to examine various courses of action.

At one extreme, he could "tell the boss to shove it."

Advantage: It is easy to do, and he gets revenge.

Disadvantage: He will have to look for a new job, probably for lower pay.

At the other extreme, he could make the more mature choice of taking a positive attitude and working hard, coming in on time, and so on.

Advantage: The boss will appreciate the improvement, take him off probation, and maybe even give him a raise.

Disadvantage: "The company will get extra mileage out of me when they've already screwed me once," plus he gets no revenge.

The therapist of course will encourage the latter choice, praising the patient (if he takes this choice) that it is, in the long run, more "manly" to do well and to have a stable life (especially if he has a family to support) than to settle for the childish satisfaction of "telling off" a boss.

It should be fairly clear from this example how this approach would be effective only at the milder end of the antisocial personality disorder spectrum. The career criminal, the psychopath, and the Ponzi-scheme scam artist are most unlikely to respond to treatment of this sort. Favorable responses depend first on the acknowledgment of fault—an element not in the true psychopath's life schema. Also, the Beck and Freeman approach, especially when applied to noninstitutionalized persons, would be more effective in antisocial patients of the predominantly impulsive type (high in Factor II traits) than in those with high Factor I traits.

The literature on the psychotherapeutic treatment of institutionalized offenders is extensive but confusing and must be read with a careful eye because of conflicting use of terms such as antisocial, sociopathic, and psychopathic. Some British writers refer to *antisocials* across the board as *psychopaths;* others restrict the term, as we have done here, to the narrower group with high PCL-R scores.

The Therapeutic Community

A favored treatment approach with institutionalized offenders, violent and nonviolent, is the therapeutic community. This multimodal treatment involves different types of group therapies, some individual cognitive therapy, and skills training; the latter enhances self-esteem and improves job opportunities after release, which will enable the patient to earn a steady livelihood and to gain self-respect.

The therapeutic community model arose in response to changes occurring in the British psychiatric hospitals after World War II. The therapeutic community model is generally used in the treatment of severe, institutionalized offenders (Dolan 1998). Various programs based on the therapeutic community model are now in use. Some embody the original core tenets of permissiveness, communalism, democratization, and reality confrontation, as in Britain's Henderson Hospital for social rehabilitation (Dolan and Coid 1993). Other programs rely on modifications when a greater sense of hierarchy and a more authoritarian atmosphere are needed. The latter approach is aimed at substance abusers and is favored by institutions in the United States. In their review of the success rates in outcome studies from Henderson Hospital spanning 8 months to 5 years, Dolan and Coid (1993) noted nonrecidivism rates (as the common success measure) of 19%–61%.

In 1962, Grendon Prison was opened in the United Kingdom, offering a therapeutic community approach to the treatment of nonpsychopathic recidivist offenders with moderate to severe personality disorders. There, the inmates had to be willing to cooperate with the regimen and were "voluntary" (free to return to ordinary prison on request). Grendon has had the lowest rate of in-prison offenses of any secure establishment.

The therapeutic community model is built around a five-step program: recognition, motivation (expression of a desire to change), understanding, insight, and testing (putting into practice new ways of coping). The success rate among offenders is not uniform. In one study, those remaining in the program longer than 9 months, for example, had a better success rate (71%) than the average rate of 41% (Dolan 1997). In another study from Henderson Hospital, patients accepted for therapeutic community were compared with others who were either not accepted or refused. Recidivism rates were lower (33%) among those accepting therapeutic community than in the untreated patients (52%). Of those who stayed with the program more than a year, only 20% relapsed. The caveat here is that those who persevered may have had more prosocial (less psychopathic) personalities to begin with and thus belonged to a prognostically better subgroup.

Therapeutic community programs appear to benefit suitable patients in several ways. The treatment may strengthen self-esteem, foster independence, heighten the level of one's moral sense, and promote conformity in attitude with respect to social norms (McCord and Sanchez 1982). The patients in the McCord study, although called *psychopaths* in the report, probably were patients with antisocial personality disorder who would not be labeled psychopaths by PCL-R standards. Also, the level of anxiety and depression may be reduced (Dolan et al. 1992), sensitivity to the feelings of others may be enhanced, progress toward developing an internal locus of control may be made (Genders and Player 1995), and a tendency to violence may be diminished (Cooke 1989).

The general consensus is that structured, behavioral, cognitive-behavioral, skills oriented, and multimodal measures, based on social learning theories, have a more beneficial effect on antisociality than do other modes of treatment (Lösel 1998). Successful programs ideally include modules that improve self-control, self-critical thinking, victim awareness, anger management, problem-solving in the interpersonal realm, vocational training, and non-criminal attitudes (Andrews et al. 1990).

These recommendations regarding the therapeutic community and related programs have limitations, particularly when applied to psychopaths meeting stringent PCL-R criteria. In the Wiltwyck-Lyman study, based on work with psychopathic boys, for example, the effects of the therapeutic community seemed promising at 1-year follow-up. But in the long-term follow-up, the levels of criminal recidivism and alcoholism were about the same as in the non–therapeutic community–treated boys (McCord and Sanchez 1982). Recidivism was 70% in both the therapeutic community and the traditional/discipline groups in this population (Craft et al. 1964).

In an intriguing study by Marnie Rice and her co-workers in Ontario, Canada, psychopathic offenders not only failed to show improvement following immersion in a therapeutic community program but actually relapsed to a higher degree than did their untreated counterparts (Rice 1997; Rice et al. 1992): 77% versus 55% in the untreated group. Offenders with PCL-R scores less than 25, in contrast, relapsed less: 22% versus 38% in the untreated group. Rice suggested as an explanation for this paradoxical finding that the nonpsychopathic persons learned how to be more empathic and concerned about others, as an outgrowth of their therapeutic community treatment. The psychopathic individuals with PCL-R scores greater than 29 "simply learned how to *appear* more empathic. They used the information from their therapeutic community programs to manipulate and deceive others in a more clever way than they knew how to do before" (Rice 1997, p. 415). As for violent recidivism, the PCL-R emerged as the best predictor and proved better than any combination of other criminal history variables.

The Factor I traits single out the most treatment-resistant psychopathy in antisocial persons who might be receptive to therapeutic community treatment. For the latter approach to work, or for any treatment modality to work, within the domain of antisociality, there are some minimal characterological requirements: a capacity, even if initially meager, for collaboration and self-reflection and an ability to endure and to benefit from criticism. In the therapeutic community situation, the patients are antisocial offenders remanded to institutions. The institutional staff must respect the dignity and rights of the residents; the residents must respect the humanness and worthiness of the staff. This was the philosophy of Thomas Main, who coined the term *therapeutic community* in 1946—a community in which the residents actively participate in their own treatment and in setting the rules and regulations for harmonious living within the institution. All this is antithetical to the mind-set of the psychopathic person, especially of the high Factor I type. Presumably, the failure of the psychopathic boys to sustain improvement in the Wiltwyck-Lyman therapeutic community program reflects a similar personality deficit that creates, most of the time, an insuperable roadblock in the path of therapeutic progress.

Child psychiatrists have begun to recognize psychopathy-in-embryo in certain children and adolescents; namely, those with "callous/unemotional" traits (Christian et al. 1997). The presence of callous/unemotional traits, combined with serious conduct problems, marks out a "unique subgroup of antisocial children… who correspond more closely to adult psychopathy" (p. 233). Closer attention to these Factor I traits, assessed according to norms relevant to juveniles, may help us to distinguish more effectively those young persons with antisociality who are most likely from those who are least likely to benefit from the various treatment approaches currently available.

Antisocial Persons Who Commit Sexual Offenses

Not all persons who commit sexual offenses also meet criteria for antisocial personality disorder. But the nature of such offenses points to, at the very least, a circumscribed area of antisocial behavior, often within the context of some other disturbances of personality. These offenses may range from exhibitionism and "date-rape" to stranger-rape and serial sexual homicide. In regard to paraphilia alone, Abel et al. (1988) cited some 21 varieties, including incestuous and nonincestuous pedophilia, sadism or masochism, frotteurism, and obscene telephone calling. They showed that 9 of 10 paraphiliacs indulged in more than one pattern (often two to four or more). Some sex offenders (almost all of whom are men) whose pattern includes voyeurism or fetishism, which is not dangerous, also commit sexual acts that do adversely affect others.

Abel et al. (1992) reviewed extensively the literature on treatment of paraphilias, pointing to the discouragingly poor success rate until the advent of direct behavioral interventions in the 1970s. Earlier, aversive techniques were emphasized, in the hope of decreasing a patient's arousal to inappropriate stimuli (e.g., children). Training in social and occupational skills has been added to most treatment programs in recent years to address the low self-esteem and meager social skills that otherwise tend to keep sex offenders frozen in their abnormal patterns. As with other forms of antisociality, a capacity for accepting responsibility, for openness about one's behavior, and for remorse is a precondition for favorable outcome. Those lacking such qualities (most habitual sex offenders) are mostly beyond the reach of currently available therapies. Persons committing multiple rapes of strangers or serial sexual homicide (or sadism without homicide)—acts that have more to do with power and violence than with sex per se—usually show antisocial personality disorder proper, or psychopathy, and have a particularly poor prognosis. Among institutionalized (including incarcerated) sex offenders of the more severe type, recidivism remains high (Quinsey et al. 1998).

Currently, the most effective treatment for men with deviant sexual behavior (primarily the less dangerous paraphiliacs) is a combined approach using cognitive-behavioral therapy (usually with skills training) focusing on overcoming abnormal attitudes and fears concerning women and hormonal pharmacotherapy. The latter involves the use of medications that lower libido, such as antiandrogens (e.g., medroxyprogesterone; Meyer et al. 1992); drugs that antagonize the action of testosterone (e.g., cyproterone; Bradford and Pawlak 1993); or drugs that selectively suppress pituitary-gonadal function (e.g., triptorelin; Rösler and Witztum 1998). Triptorelin (not yet available in the United States) has the advantage that it can be administered intramuscularly once a month.

Conclusion

The term *antisociality* as used here was chosen for its wide coverage, answering to the entire range of antisocial behaviors, from isolated acts occurring during a comparatively brief span over the life course to unequivocal instances of antisocial personality disorder and psychopathy, with or without violence. In the sexual sphere, the spectrum ranges from date-rape, voyeurism, or exhibitionism to rape of strangers and, finally, to serial sexual homicide preceded by prolonged torture.

From the standpoint of prognosis and treatability, *psychopathy* as redefined by Hare and colleagues is a tighter concept than DSM's antisocial personality disorder, offering more reliable clues to outcome and amenability to treatment than does the current definition of antisocial personality disorder. Persons with high scores on the PCL-R, in whom psychopathy is diagnosed (in contrast to the presence of a few psychopathic traits), almost never experience themselves as in need of psychiatric help, the very notion of which they look down on with contempt. Thus, they situate themselves beyond the pale of psychiatry as a healing profession. Also, many nonpsychopathic persons with antisocial personality disorder (or with some antisocial traits) will drop their antisocial ways as they reach mid-life, but this tends not to happen with psychopathic persons.

Recent neurophysiological research is helping to bolster the concept and the clinical usefulness of psychopathy, establishing correlations (in evoked potential and in neuroanatomical studies) between high PCL-R scores and functional brain differences. The broader and less specific concept of antisocial personality disorder (of which psychopathy is a subset) would not yield as robust correlations. Further research is necessary to delineate whether the secondary psychopathy apparently stemming from severe early abuse (Porter 1996) is distinguishable from primary (or what appears to be innate) psychopathy, or whether the same brain changes can occur—and become "hard-wired"—following postnatal trauma.

The concept of *sadism* needs further research as well. Many persons with antisocial personality disorder or psychopathy subject others, especially intimates, to the grievous maltreatment we call sadism. As with the two major conditions, sadism itself comes in two "flavors": psychological (repeatedly humiliating and degrading others) and physical (subjecting others to torture) (Stone 1998). Either form has a poor prognosis: sadism is notoriously resistant to treatment. Many persons who become sadistic were themselves the victims of caregiver abuse or neglect in early life; we need to know whether there are, in some cases at least, genetic or constitutional predispositions to behave sadistically. Here, the study of psychopathic persons who have not been subjected to childhood trauma yet become sadistic may yield important clues.

In my forensic work, I have begun to find an impressive correlation between the PCL-R item *criminal versatility* and high scores on the PCL-R in general. This is not surprising because many psychopathic individuals carry out a wide variety of offenses and are arrested for crimes in half a dozen different categories. Forensic patients who are clearly psychotic usually have a history of injuring or killing someone, often a relative, in an uncharacteristic and impulsive act, when under great emotional stress, and in the absence of a previous record of antisocial behavior. Their PCL-R scores are at the opposite end of the range, generally less than 10. Men are much more apt to be antisocial or psychopathic than are women. The women in forensic hospitals or even prisons often show borderline personality disorder characteristics with antisocial features (or full comorbid antisocial personality disorder). Women with high PCL-R scores are uncommon. This may help account for their better long-term outcome, compared with male patients released from forensic institutions (Stone 1999).

Favorable prognosis within the realm of antisociality thus inheres to persons sufficiently free of psychopathic features as *not* to meet PCL-R diagnostic criteria. It is not yet easy to predict which nonpsychopathic persons who become patients (in regular or forensic hospitals or other facilities) will improve significantly in response to therapeutic interventions and which will improve, despite or without help, just through maturation and aging. Dynamic therapies have little place in the treatment of antisociality, apart from some malignant narcissism in persons who have enough motivation, self-awareness, honesty, and perseverance to attempt analytically oriented therapy.

Even cognitive-behavioral therapy, which is often useful in institutions dedicated to the treatment of antisocial patients, is only occasionally successful in extramural settings because of the dishonesty typical of this patient group and their tendency not to comply with suggestions, skills-training programs, limit-setting, and (when indicated) medications recommended by a therapist.

Compliance with medications makes the difference between treatable and nontreatable sex offenders (especially of the paraphilic type), given the importance of pharmacotherapy in this group. The jurist Nigel Walker (1991) offered a typology of sexual offenders: 1) those responding to "chance" situations that are sexually tempting, 2) those who "follow inclinations" (e.g., child molesters who apply for work in day-care centers), 3) those who seek opportunity, and 4) those who make opportunity. He considers the latter two types unconditionally dangerous. They usually meet criteria for psychopathy. Walker argued for the extended segregation of such offenders (repeat offenders have a very high rate of recidivism). But he recognized that the psychiatric profession, although its predictive abilities in the forensic area have improved over the past 20 years, cannot predict with 100% accuracy which offenders might never have relapsed had they been released and which offenders are most likely to. The recommendation for extended confinement, therefore, inevitably leads to the incorrect limitation of freedom of a few to protect the community from the many who would cause further harm. Walker argued that society owes to the segregated sex offenders a humane and reasonably pleasant environment to compensate for the sacrifice of freedom (on the part of those who unbeknownst to us might not have reoffended) in the interests of society. One of the heavier burdens of psychiatrists who work in the area of antisociality in general and sex offender treatment in particular is the obligation to complete ever more sophisticated studies, including long-term follow-up studies, so that each generation of psychiatrists will make more accurate judgments about treatability, about prognosis, and thus, in relation to serious and violent offenders, about whom to retain and whom to eventually release.

References

Abel GG, Becker JV, Cunningham-Rathner J, et al: Multiple paraphilic diagnoses among sex offenders. Bulletin of the American Academy of Psychiatry and Law 16:153–168, 1988

Abel GG, Osborn CA, Anthony D, et al: Current treatments of paraphiliacs. Annual Review of Sex Research 3:255–290, 1992

American Psychiatric Association: Diagnostic and Statistical Manual of Mental Disorders, 3rd Edition. Washington, DC, American Psychiatric Association, 1980

American Psychiatric Association: Diagnostic and Statistical Manual of Mental Disorders, 3rd Edition, Revised. Washington, DC, American Psychiatric Association, 1987

American Psychiatric Association: Diagnostic and Statistical Manual of Mental Disorders, 4th Edition. Washington, DC, American Psychiatric Association, 1994

Andrews DA, Zinger I, Hoge RD, et al: Does correctional treatment work? a clinically relevant and psychologically informed meta-analysis. Criminology 28:369–404, 1990

Beck AT, Freeman A: Cognitive Therapy of Personality Disorders. New York, Guilford, 1990

Bradford JMW, Pawlak A: Double-blind placebo crossover study of cyproterone acetate in the treatment of the paraphilias. Arch Sex Behav 22:383–402, 1993

Christian RE, Frick PJ, Hill NL, et al: Psychopathy and conduct problems in children, II: implications for subtyping children with conduct problems. J Am Acad Child Adolesc Psychiatry 36:233–241, 1997

Clarkin JF, Yeomans FE, Kernberg OF: Psychotherapy for Borderline Personality. New York, Wiley, 1999

Cleckley H: The Mask of Sanity. St. Louis, MO, CV Mosby, 1941

Cloninger CR: A unified biosocial theory of personality and its role in the development of anxiety states. Psychiatric Developments 3:167–226, 1986

Cloninger CR, Svrakic DM, Przybeck TR: A psychobiological model of temperament and character. Arch Gen Psychiatry 50:975–990, 1993

Cooke DJ: Containing violent prisoners: an analysis of the Barlinnie Special Unit. British Journal of Criminology 29:129–143, 1989

Craft M, Stephenson G, Granger C: A controlled study of authoritarian and self-governing regimes with adolescent psychopaths. Am J Orthopsychiatry 34:543–554, 1964

Dolan B: A community-based therapeutic community: the Henderson Hospital, in A Community Based Therapeutic Community for Offenders. Edited by Cullen E, Jones L, Woodward R. Chichester, England, Wiley, 1997, pp 47–74

Dolan B: Therapeutic community treatment for severe personality disorders, in Psychopathy: Antisocial, Criminal and Violent Behavior. Edited by Millon T, Simonsen E, Birket-Smith M, et al. New York, Guilford, 1998, pp 407–430

Dolan B, Coid J: Therapeutic community approaches, in Psychopathic and Antisocial Personality Disorders. Edited by Dolan B, Coid J. London, England, Gaskell, 1993, pp 146–180

Dolan B, Evans C, Wilson J: Therapeutic community treatment for personality disordered adults: changes in neurotic symptomatology on follow-up. Int J Soc Psychiatry 38:243–250, 1992

Franke D: The Torture Doctor. New York, Hawthorne Press, 1975

Gabbard G: Psychodynamic Psychotherapy in Clinical Practice. Washington, DC, American Psychiatric Press, 1994

Genders E, Player E: Grendon: A Study of a Therapeutic Prison. Oxford, England, Clarendon, 1995

Hare RD: Psychopathy: a clinical construct whose time has come. Criminal Justice and Behavior 23:25–54, 1995

Hare RD, McPherson LM: Violent and aggressive behavior by criminal psychopaths. Int J Law Psychiatry 7:329–337, 1984

Hare RD, Hart SD, Harpur TJ: Psychopathy and the DSM-IV criteria for antisocial personality disorder. J Abnorm Psychol 100:391–398, 1991

Harpur TJ, Hare RD, Hakstian AR: Two-factor conceptualization of psychopathy: construct validity and assessment implications. J Consult Clin Psychol 1:6–17, 1989

Harris GT, Rice ME, Quinsey VL: Psychopathy as a taxon: evidence that psychopaths are a discrete class. J Consult Clin Psychol 62:387–397, 1994

Hart SD, Hare RD, Forth AE: Psychopathy as a risk marker for violence: development and validation of a screening version of the Revised Psychopathy Checklist, in Violence and Mental Disorder. Edited by Monahan J, Steadman H. Chicago, IL, University of Chicago Press, 1994, pp 81–98

Havill A: The Mother, the Son, and the Socialite: The True Story of a Mother-Son Crime Spree. New York, St Martin's Press, 1999

Hemphill JF, Templeman R, Wong S, et al: Psychopathy and crime: recidivism and criminal careers, in Psychopathy. Edited by Cooke DJ, Forth AE, Hare RD. Dordrecht, The Netherlands, Kluwer, 1998, pp 375–399

Huesman LR, Eron LD, Lefkowitz MM, et al: Stability of aggression over time and generations. Dev Psychol 20:1120–1134, 1984

Kernberg HAVE: Aggression in Personality Disorders & Perversions. New Haven, CT, Yale University Press, 1992

af Klinteberg B: Biology and personality: findings from a longitudinal project, in Psychopathy. Edited by Cooke DJ, Forth AE, Hare RD. Dordrecht, The Netherlands, Kluwer, 1998, pp 139–160

Kohlberg L: The Psychology of Moral Development. New York, Harper & Row, 1984

Kraepelin E: Psychiatrie: Ein Lehrbuch für Studierende und Ärzte. Leipzig, Germany, JA Barth, 1915, pp 1973–2116

Lösel F: Treatment and management of psychopaths, in Psychopathy: Theory, Research and Implications for Society. Edited by Cooke D, Forth A, Hare R. Dordrecht, The Netherlands, Kluwer, 1998, pp 303–354

McCord W, Sanchez J: The Wiltwyck-Lyman project: a 25 year follow-up study of milieu therapy, in The Psychopath and Milieu Therapy: A Longitudinal Study. Edited by McCord W. New York, Academic Press, 1982, pp 229–296

McGuire C, Norton C: Perfect Victim: A True Story of Riveting Psychological Intensity by the Assistant D.A. Who Prosecuted the Captor of the "Girl in the Box." New York, Arbor House/William & Morrow, 1988

McGuire M, Troisi A: Darwinian Psychiatry. Oxford, England, Oxford University Press, 1998

McGuire M, Fawzy FI, Spar JE, et al: Altruism and mental disorders. Ethology & Sociobiology 15:299–321, 1994

Meloy JR: The Psychopathic Mind. Northvale, NJ, Jason Aronson, 1988

Meyer WJ III, Cole C, Emory E: Depo-provera treatment for sex offending behavior: an evaluation of outcome. Bull Am Acad Psychiatry Law 20:249–259, 1992

Michaud S, Aynesworth H: The Only Living Witness. New York, Simon & Schuster, 1983

Myers WA: A case history of a man who made obscene telephone calls and practiced frotteurism, in Perversions and Near Perversions. Edited by Fogel GI, Myers WA. New Haven, CT, Yale University Press, 1991, pp 100–123

Porter S: Without conscience or without active conscience? The etiology of psychopathy revisited. Aggression and Violent Behavior 1:179–189, 1996

Quinsey VL, Harris GT, Rice ME, et al: Sex offenders, in Violent Offenders: Appraising & Managing Risk. Washington, DC, American Psychological Association, 1998, pp 119–137

Rice ME: Violent offender research and implication for the criminal justice system. Am Psychol 52:414–423, 1997

Rice ME, Harris GT, Cormier CA: An evaluation of maximum security therapeutic community for psychopaths and other disordered offenders. Law Hum Behav 16:399–412, 1992

Robins LN, Tipp J, Przybeck T: Antisocial personality, in Psychiatric Disorders in America. Edited by Robins LN, Regier DA. New York, Macmillan, 1991, pp 258–290

Rösler A, Witztum E: Treatment of men with paraphilia with a long-acting analogue of gonadotropin-releasing hormone. N Engl J Med 338:416–422, 1998

Sereny G: Cries Unheard: Why Children Kill—The Story of Mary Bell. New York, Henry Holt, 1998

Stone MH: The personalities of murderers: the importance of psychopathy and sadism, in Psychopathology and Violent Crime. Edited by Skodol AE. Washington, DC, American Psychiatric Press, 1998, pp 29–52

Stone MH: Long term follow-up of insanity acquittees released from a maximum security forensic hospital: lecture June 3, 1999, Florence, Italy for the Società Italiana di Psichiatria Penitenziaria

Taubman B: The Preppy Murder Trial. New York, St. Martin's Press, 1988

Walker N: Dangerous mistakes. Br J Psychiatry 158:752–757, 1991

Chapter 5

Cognitive Therapy for Personality Disorders

Peter Tyrer, M.D.
Kate Davidson, Ph.D.

Cognitive therapy was developed by Beck (1967) as a means of treating depressive disorders. It has subsequently been developed to include the treatment of anxiety in all its forms (Beck et al. 1985), hypochondriasis or health anxiety (Warwick 1989; Warwick et al. 1996), substance use (Nishith et al. 1997), and schizophrenia (Kingdon et al. 1994). Indeed, some cynics have suggested that there is no psychiatric disorder for which cognitive therapy cannot be given because it appears to be a universal treatment. In some ways, this is not surprising; cognitive therapy comprises a set of standard techniques that change errors or biases in cognitions of psychiatric patients with mental state disorders. There is no reason that such errors or biases should be confined to only certain disorders; thus, on a priori grounds, there is no reason that cognitive therapy should not be used to manage personality disorders. Indeed, because many people with depression, anxiety, and other disorders suitable for treatment with cognitive therapy also have a personality disorder, therapists commonly use cognitive techniques when dealing with abnormal attitudes and behavior created by personality disorders.

For example, in one case study of the use of cognitive therapy to treat dysthymic disorder in a university student, the patient "engaged repeatedly in self-damaging acts, cut his arms and abdomen with a razor, showed intense and inappropriate anger, could not bear being alone, and engaged in impulsive behavior such as driving his motorbike in a reckless fashion" (Blackburn and Davidson 1995, p. 196). The techniques of cognitive therapy directed at the impulsive, harmful behavior were not considered in principle to be significantly different from the techniques of cognitive-behavioral therapy used to address symptoms and behavior of depression. Therefore, cognitive therapy was used to try to modify the impulsivity (Blackburn and Davidson 1995). One of the main differences between personality disorders (Axis II) and mental state disorders (Axis I) is that personality is more intrinsic and ingrained, so it is more difficult to understand maladaptive perceptions of the self and of relationships to individuals and to the world. Therefore, it is not appropriate to transfer the techniques of cognitive therapy directly to personality disorders as if they were another group of mental state disorders.

There are important similarities and differences between cognitive therapy in personality disorders and cognitive therapy in mental state disorders, and these are shown in Table 5–1. Throughout this chapter, *cognitive therapy* could be regarded as including cognitive-behavioral therapy because most cognitive therapists do not adopt the pure distinction between thinking and behavior, which at times has been regarded as the essential feature differentiating cognitive and behavior therapy.

Many other treatments are linked to cognitive therapy, either closely or distantly, but they are not discussed here. These include interpersonal psychotherapy, other forms of brief psychotherapy, analytic or quasi-analytic therapies, and cognitive analytic therapy. The evidence to date does not indicate that any of these therapies are less or more superior to cognitive therapy in the treatment of borderline personality disorder (Shea 1991; Stone 1990). Also, dialectical behavior therapy is not discussed here, but it is sufficiently distinct from cognitive therapy, despite its origins, to be regarded as a separate type of treatment. No comparisons between cognitive therapy and dialectical behavior therapy have been made, and their relative worth can be only speculative. There is also concern that a comparison of the efficacy of these different approaches may sometimes select the wrong outcomes, because an overpreoccupation with improvement of symptoms is not necessarily the best way to determine success in treating personality disorders (Benjamin 1997). However, because comparison among psychotherapies for personality disorder is relatively uncharted territory, and evidence-based recommendations do not yet exist,

Table 5–1. Differences in cognitive therapy between mental state and personality disorders

	Mental state disorders	Personality disorders
Length of treatment	3–4 months	9 months or longer
Pace of treatment	Brisk	Variable, at patient's pace
Problem time scale	Here and now	Here and now and lifetime
Therapeutic relationship	Collaborative	Collaborative with clear patient-therapist boundaries
Problem content	Patient's world; present and future	Patient's world; past, present, and future; therapeutic relationship
Problem focus	Behavior; cognition; emotion	Behavior; cognition; emotion; therapeutic relationship
Emphasis in intervention	Automatic thoughts	Behavior schemas
Homework	Automatic thoughts; data collection	Behavioral; data collection; reworking of beliefs
Scientific method	Experimental	Experimental
Learning model	Maladaptive learning	Maladaptive learning or failure to learn through lack of appropriate opportunity
Openness	Explicit	Explicit; rule bound

Source. From Davidson K: *Cognitive Therapy for Personality Disorders: A Clinician's Guide.* Oxford, England, Butterworth-Heinemann, 2000. Reprinted with permission of Butterworth-Heinemann Publishers, a division of Reed Educational & Professional Publishing Ltd.

different types of psychotherapy cannot be compared usefully in this chapter.

Theoretical Rationale for Cognitive Therapy

The major theorists behind the use of cognitive therapy for personality disorders are Beck and Freeman (1990) and Young (1990,

1994). Because personality is so much more ingrained than the clinical symptoms of mental disorders, it is not appropriate to regard personality disorders as conditions in which a few persistent errors in cognition could be responsible for a large part of the abnormal features. Instead, fundamental core beliefs, or schemas, which combine a knowledge base and specific rules, are thought to generate a range of maladaptive thoughts and behavior. Because these thoughts and behaviors are intrinsic to the individual, they are not always recognized as alien or unwanted; they are either accepted as part of normal functioning or projected to others so that the individual decides that the fault lies elsewhere. Hence the motivation for change that is so important in the success of psychological therapies is often much less evident in people with personality disorders than in other conditions. An additional problem is that because the conditions are long-standing, it is very difficult for some individuals to find a reference point from the past when functioning was closer to normal. Under these circumstances, a standard cognitive technique, such as challenging the basis of assumptions about a symptom or behavior, is correspondingly more difficult.

Beck and colleagues (1990) regard personality traits as evolutionary strategies that preserve survival and reproduction and are therefore important in the process of Darwinian natural selection. Traits, according to this model, lead to programmed behaviors involving cognitive, affective, motivational, and arousal processes, and they generally produce a pattern of stereotyped behaviors that were biologically advantageous in primitive societies. However, because the environment in which humans now find themselves has developed so dramatically over the past few millennia, these behaviors do not always match the environmental requirements. Mismatch leads to personality disorder, a prime example of an inappropriate fit between person and environment and, most prominently, the social environment.

The programmed behaviors are directly linked to the schemas, which cover the whole range of personal activity subserving emotion, drive, and choice. The cognitive schemas are not unopposed and sometimes are forced into uneasy compromises. Beck and colleagues (1990) suggested that personality disorders are the consequence of an inappropriate and maladaptive interaction between the cognitive schemas and those schemas concerning affect, motivation, action, and control, and these specific interactions lead to the specific patterns of thinking, emotion, or behavior that are characteristic of personality disorders. This theory has been developed further by Arntz (1994, 1999; Arntz et al. 1999) into a more tightly formulated structure that matches formulation and assessment of personality disorders, particularly the borderline group, in the most effective way.

The Practice of Cognitive Therapy With Personality Disorders

In the United Kingdom, most people are treated in a publicly funded service, the National Health Service, in which treatment is free at the point of delivery. It is genuinely free and not paid for by insurance or any other agency. Therefore, concern over rationing treatments that are resource intensive is great, and limited resources are available for psychotherapeutic treatments in general. Those treatments that are recommended tend to be brief and focused, such as cognitive-behavioral therapy. Treatment also needs to be given to all people in society, including many with limited literary and intellectual skills, so adaptations may be necessary for this population. Most people coming for cognitive-behavioral therapy for personality disorder in the United Kingdom have had no previous exposure to psychotherapy, and this also must be taken into account.

In developing a treatment protocol for the cognitive treatment of personality disorders, we have attempted to limit treatment to no longer than 9 months. Nonetheless, all essential elements are covered (Davidson, in press), and the following features are included:

- Attention to engagement by means of the principle of collaborative empiricism, a fundamental approach in cognitive therapy that enables psychotherapeutic treatment of disorders that normally would be thought of as difficult to treat with psychotherapy, such as chronic schizophrenia, to have considerable success (Tarrier et al. 1999).

- A full and open formulation of the patient's problems. This formulation is shared with the patient and guides treatment. Through this, the cognitive approach allows patients to develop a better understanding of how earlier life experiences may have influenced their extreme views of themselves and others and resulted in the identified problems in later life. The interpersonal problems and behavioral difficulties that are so common can be likewise understood and modified as new ways of perceiving, thinking, and behaving can be tested out within the relatively safe environment of therapy.
- Agreement of goals of therapy, with reduction of self-harm and harm to others given the highest priority.
- Addressing personality problems in terms of environmental "fit." Alternative ways of behaving and thinking are explored as being a better "fit."
- Treatment that focuses on identifying maladaptive cognitions and behaviors (including interpersonal difficulties) and changing these to more appropriate ways of thinking and behaving. Behavioral experiments are used to test changes in long-established schemas.

Because many patients with personality disorders are very difficult to engage in therapy, it may take several weeks before these principles are accepted. A significant part of the engagement is orienting patients to the treatment by a careful assessment and formulation of their problems and the establishment of agreed-on goals to be achieved in therapy.

Effectiveness of Cognitive Therapy for Personality Disorders

We examined the effectiveness of cognitive therapy in borderline and antisocial personality disorders by closely evaluating single cases (Davidson and Tyrer 1996). This process involved the use of the treatment protocol described earlier in this chapter (Davidson, in press), which includes elements of Beck's cognitive model of psychopathology, the schema-focused therapy of Young, and some skill elements from dialectical behavior therapy (Linehan 1992). Because it can be inappropriate to be too prescriptive in this treatment, each individual seen was assessed, and an individual formulation was made, which guided the treatment plan. A treatment plan was formed after the patient identified the problems that created most of the difficulties with regard to personality functioning. Initially, treatment consisted of a block of 10 sessions, each lasting 1 hour, at approximately weekly intervals. After this time, treatment progress was reviewed regularly and, if necessary, appropriate adjustments made to the treatment plan. Because of the disorganization created by personality disturbance in these people, we believed that rigid times for each appointment were not necessarily appropriate. Although weekly sessions were planned, longer periods between sessions were allowed to permit individuals the time to practice new ways of behaving and thinking before moving on to the next phase of treatment.

Single-case methodology (Hersen and Barlow 1976) with the classic AB design was used (Peck 1992), and data were analyzed by interrupted time-series analysis (ITSACORR) (Crosbie 1993). This conservative program reduces false-positive results (to a minimum) and is suitable for data collected consecutively over a short time. Problems were assessed with an adapted form of the Personal Questionnaire Rapid Scaling Technique (PQRST) (Mulhall 1976), in which patients were asked to rate the degree to which a specific problem was creating difficulty. This rating was converted into an 11-point numerical scale: a score of 10 indicated no problems, and a score of 0 indicated maximum distress or problem behavior. Although this approach has not been commonly used in the assessment of personality disorders, it was thought to be appropriate here because each of the three problems had been identified specifically, and the rating system was fully understood. Although self-ratings are not always satisfactory in assessing personality disorders, the advantages of frequent ratings (daily assessment) were considerable, and because each problem had been identified by the patient as personally important, it was more likely to be reliably rated and ensured that both assessment and treatment progress were attuned. This provided a highly specific and sensitive measure of progress in treatment.

Over a 1-year period, 12 patients referred by general practitioners and local psychiatric services were seen—4 with antisocial personality disorder and 8 with borderline personality disorder diagnosed with the Munich Diagnostic Checklist Criteria (Hiller et al. 1991). Two patients were not fully entered into the study because they were unable to travel to appointments due to changes in their circumstances; of the remaining 10 patients, 2 discontinued treatment before adequate data for evaluation were available. Of the remaining 8 patients, only 1 failed to show significant progress during the course of treatment that lasted up to 9 months. A case example of one of the patients treated, a man who had been in prison for drug-violence offenses and had been violent toward his wife, follows.

> On entry into the pilot study, the patient, an unemployed 44-year-old man, had been frequently violent toward his wife, had been charged with assaulting another man, and was awaiting sentencing. Although not dependent on alcohol, he had episodes of heavy drinking during which he could not remember what he was doing, and on these occasions, he frequently assaulted his wife. The three core problems were identified as
>
> 1. His relationship with his wife
> 2. His feelings toward others (e.g., friendly, hostile)
> 3. A desire to "feel calm"

The results of the treatment are shown in Table 5–2; a somewhat unusual immediate effect of cognitive therapy on all three key problem areas was seen, although because of the conservative nature of the ITSACORR program, only one of these was deemed to be significant. The major change in treatment occurred early after the baseline assessments and was quite dramatic.

> The patient had a dismissive and negative attitude toward his wife at the onset of therapy. He considered her to be a weak and spineless person who had no opinions of her own and so she was both bullied and despised. He was asked to reexamine this view and determine whether there were alternative explanations. In a therapy session, this was discussed with his wife, and he was somewhat surprised to discover that her views were quite different. In the relative safety of the clinical session, she

Table 5–2. Mean weekly scores on three key problems from a case study of a patient with antisocial personality disorder treated with cognitive therapy

	Relationship with wife	Feelings toward others	"Feeling calm"
	Before treatment		
Week 1	2.6	3.1	3.6
Week 2	1.7	3.1	2.9
	After treatment		
Week 3	5.4	6.3	6.4
Week 4	7.4	8.0	8.6
Week 5	6.0	6.7	4.7
Week 6	5.7	4.9	5.6
Week 7	5.7	6.4	8.0
Week 8	7.0	7.0	7.7
Week 9	7.4	7.0	6.9

Note. All scores on a 0–10 scale, with lower scores indicating greater problems.

Difference between baseline and treatment ratings: relationship with wife: $F = 3.41$; $df = 2.60$; $P = 0.04$; feelings toward others: $F = 1.84$, not significant; feeling calm: $F = 2.82$, not significant.

Source. Adapted from Davidson and Tyrer 1996.

described being frightened of him when he was angry, particularly after he had been drinking. To avoid the possibility of conflict, she tried her best to be accommodating and to please him in every way because she was frightened that he would hit her if she made "mistakes." His wife was involved in three subsequent sessions (the therapy allows involvement of significant others when indicated) to evaluate the specific components of this relationship; his wife also was seen individually. The patient was asked the following challenging questions: What sort of wife and relationship did he want? Was it in his interests to "make" her incompetent? What could he do to improve their relationship?

Through guided discovery, he became aware of the damaging nature of his attitude toward his wife and how his behavior toward her was undermining and counterproductive. It became evident that he wanted an intimate partner, was afraid of being alone, and was more aware that the marriage was threatened if he continued his behavior. They made a pact to drink less when together, he resolved not to be critical when she made errors, and her self-confidence improved. These changes were further consolidated during therapy, and he came to understand that most of the difficulties in their relationship had been created by his incorrect beliefs about his wife. The changes also led to improvements in the other two goals of treatment.

At this stage of development, this approach can only be said to show promise, and we are currently trying to evaluate it more formally in a randomized controlled trial. One of the important positive features in our case series was the low dropout rate once patients had become engaged in therapy. We also have developed this treatment further in the management of deliberate self-harm (parasuicide) in patients with personality disorders within the flamboyant cluster (ICD-10 [World Health Organization 1992] diagnoses of dissocial [antisocial], histrionic, emotionally unstable [impulsive and borderline] personality disorders); here, we formally evaluated the intervention in a randomized controlled trial. We shortened the treatment to six sessions and reinforced it with a set of treatment booklets (bibliotherapy), including some skill components of Marsha Linehan's dialectical behavior therapy. This combined treatment is called *manual-assisted cognitive-behavioral therapy* (MACT), and although it is not normally recommended to be given in six sessions, the population who self-harm are very difficult to engage in therapy. Those who fail to stay for assessment and treatment are more likely to repeat this behavior (Crawford and Wessely 1998), and any treatment given is likely to have a high dropout rate. The treatment is designed to be flexible, and therapists can use whichever elements of treatment are considered most relevant following a formulation of the patient's problems.

To detect possible effects of intervention, a population at high risk for repetition was selected. All patients included were seen after an episode of deliberate self-harm and were between ages 16 and 50, had personality disturbance within the flamboyant personality cluster, and had had at least one other episode of deliberate self-harm in the previous 12 months. Patients with a primary ICD-10 diagnosis within the organic (F0), alcohol or drug dependence (F1), or schizophrenia (F2) groups were excluded.

In this randomized controlled trial, patients were allocated to either the experimental treatment (MACT) or the treatment as usual (TAU) in each of two centers. MACT, a brief, cognitively oriented, and problem-focused therapy of between two and six sessions, is structured around a manual covering problem-solving, basic cognitive techniques to manage emotions and negative thinking, and relapse prevention strategies. Five therapists (one psychiatrist, two nurses, and two social workers) were trained in the use of the treatment to ensure that the information in the manual could be structured around the patient's current problems.

Initially, therapists gave patients the first chapter of the manual. All patients were then encouraged to use worksheets contained in the first chapter to analyze the circumstances surrounding the episode of deliberate self-harm leading to their presentation. In later sessions, the patient and the therapist selected and worked through relevant chapters from the manual to help the patient deal with specific problems that they mutually agreed were the most important in leading to the patient's self-harm acts. If the patient did not attend further therapy, the remaining five chapters were sent by post. Between sessions, patients were encouraged to practice their newly acquired skills by using problem-solving or distress tolerance techniques.

The point of allocation was immediately after baseline assessment had been completed by an independent assessor who had no contact with the clinical teams during the study and made assessments without any knowledge of the treatment received. Patients were allocated by opening sealed opaque envelopes sequentially at each center. The time to next parasuicidal act was selected as the main outcome measure because of the encouraging results of one study (Salkovskis et al. 1990), and rate of acts per month, depressive and anxiety symptoms, social function, and costs of care were secondary measures.

At follow-up, 32 patients (18 MACT, 14 TAU) were seen, and 10 patients in each group (56% MACT, 71% TAU) had a suicidal act during the 6 months. Although the main hypothesis—that there would be a delay to the next suicidal act—was only partly supported (the median time to next suicidal act was 142 days in the MACT group and 114 days in the TAU group), the rate of suicidal acts per month was lower with MACT (median 0.17/month MACT; 0.37/month TAU; $P = 0.11$), and self-rated depressive symptoms improved significantly (mean Hospital Anxiety and Depression Scale scores [Zigmond and Snaith 1983] at follow-up: 5.7 MACT; 10.1 TAU; $P = 0.03$). The treatment was given economically, involving a mean of 2.7 sessions (several patients had the MACT manual only), and the observed average cost of care was 46% less with MACT (Evans et al. 1999), mainly because more of the TAU patients had longer periods of inpatient hospital care.

These favorable results were reinforced by evidence from a substudy in which positive and negative future thinking were evaluated. Patients were seen at baseline immediately after the para-suicidal act and given a short task to determine both positive and negative thoughts about the future. They were reassessed after 6 months with the same task. Those randomized to MACT showed a significantly greater increase in positive future thinking than those allocated to TAU (Macleod et al. 1998), suggesting that cognitive changes had occurred during treatment and were maintained.

The work in this area has been expanded to a large multicenter, randomized controlled trial supported by the Medical Research Council (United Kingdom) of 500 patients in five centers in England and Scotland, which has just finished recruiting subjects.

Cognitive Therapy in Patients With Axis I and Axis II Comorbidity

Most studies have shown that the presence of personality disorder at the same time as a mental (Axis I) disorder tends to impair the outcome of treatment (Black et al. 1994; Chambless et al. 1997; Hardy et al. 1995; Patience et al. 1995; Tyrer et al. 1997), although this is not universal. However, it should be emphasized that the treatments in these studies were for the Axis I disorder and not specifically directed at the Axis II disorder. The one clear exception is obsessive-compulsive personality disorder. When cognitive therapy is given for obsessive-compulsive disorder, the outcome does not seem to be influenced if obsessive-compulsive personality disorder is also present (Dreessen et al. 1997), and the effects of the cognitive therapy on the Axis I obsessional disorder (which have independently been shown to be positive) (de Haan et al. 1997) also may extend to the personality disorder component.

Many research studies that find a worse response in people with personality disorders may not have taken enough account of the differences in symptomatology and behavior at baseline. Patients with personality disorders characteristically have more severe Axis I symptoms that last longer and cause more disruption than in those without personality disorders (Tyrer et al. 1990, 1997); unless this is taken into account, the outcomes will appear worse in those with personality disorders. When allowances are made for this, the outcomes may be even better in those with personality disorders, particularly in patients with alcohol disorders (Griggs and Tyrer 1981; Longabaugh et al. 1994).

In at least one group, those with neurotic disorders, conventional cognitive therapy for mental state disorders does not appear to be effective at the same time for personality disorders in those with Axis I and Axis II comorbidity. In a 2-year study of 210 patients with one of three DSM neurotic disorders—generalized anxiety disorder, dysthymic disorder, or panic disorder—in which cognitive therapy was compared with drug treatment (primarily antidepressants) and a self-help package, those with a comorbid personality disorder had a significantly worse outcome in the longer term when treated with cognitive therapy or self-help than those treated with drugs (Tyrer et al. 1993). Although we had independent evidence that some of the cognitive therapy was administered by less than satisfactory therapists (Kingdon et al. 1996), the results are still important to acknowledge.

If these results are replicated in other disorders, it suggests that when cognitive therapy is being administered for those with personality disorders, it should focus specifically on the personality aspects and take account of the differences between Axis I and II disorders in delivering this treatment (Table 5–1). More work must be done on the interaction between pharmacological and cognitive treatments for comorbid disorders, and although preliminary evidence suggests that they are synergistic (de Haan et al. 1997), this must not be assumed to always be the case. As in clinical practice, it is always more common to encounter comorbid rather than pure personality disorders, seen most strongly with the borderline group (Fyer et al. 1988); this subject should remain high on the research agenda.

Outcome of Patients With Comorbid Axis I and Axis II Disorders

In evaluating the outcome of borderline patients, it is important to recognize that dropout rates are high, yet outcome is relatively good. Stone (1990), on the basis of his personal experience, stated that 40% of patients drop out of treatment regardless of who is seeing them, yet two out of three "if followed long enough, eventually have a good result" (p. 281). This hypothesis has yet to be tested satisfactorily, but it is reasonable to assume that the treatment that is likely to keep the patient in contact with therapy during the period of active involvement is likely to be better than one that leads to a greater dropout rate. In deciding on the relative value of each treatment, both pharmacological and nonpharmacological, for personality disorder, dropout rates may therefore be extremely valuable.

Prediction of Future Developments in the Cognitive Treatment of Personality Disorders

Despite considerable interest in this subject over the past 10 years, the evidence base for cognitive therapy in personality disorders is still very small. Most of the studies have been done in those with borderline personality disorder, but because great variability is found in the outcome of this group (Links et al. 1998), naturalistic follow-up studies are of little value in determining the efficacy of this approach. Despite their methodological difficulties in the evaluation of those with personality disorders, randomized controlled trials are essential to establish the value of these treatment approaches, and to date none have been carried out except in the area of parasuicide.

Much more work is needed on the other groups of personality disorders in the classification system. Again, these are likely to be complicated by comorbidity issues, but apart from the obsessive-compulsive group, none of the other conditions outside the flamboyant spectrum has been studied, except in nonrandomized trials (see Sanislow and McGlashan 1998). One of the main assets of the cognitive therapeutic approach is its ability to reach patients who generally reject other psychotherapeutic approaches. It probably achieves this by spending time and effort in establishing a framework under which the therapist and subject can work comfortably and that also serves as a sounding board where the goals and form of treatment can be established (Davidson, in press). Although this time is less than with some other forms of psychotherapy, it is an important requirement that helps to keep the patient engaged when, at times in the future, the treatment takes a more rocky course. More work is needed to determine whether the challenge of dealing with the schizoid and paranoid group of personality disorders can be taken up, and the needs of the dependent and anxious group are equally strong. The evidence from the comorbid studies suggests that "standard" cognitive therapy for Axis I disorders is not sufficient to improve the personality components, and combined packages of treatment suitable for treating both mental state and personality components of the treatment are probably needed.

Comparative studies among the different psychological treatments now available for personality disorder are also needed. The history of medicine suggests that whenever many treatments are available for a condition, with the value of each loudly proclaimed by its advocates, the likelihood that very few of them are really effective is strong. The current approach to the treatment jungle, nicely summarized as the ABCDE approach by Stone (1990), in which the therapist looks at analytical therapy (A), behavior therapy (B), cognitive therapy (C), and drug therapy (D) and then picks and chooses to create an eclectic therapy (E), might be the best approach in the state of current confusion, but it is of no long-term value. Where cognitive therapy will stand when it emerges from the jungle is difficult to predict, but we venture to suggest that it will still be standing as a valid treatment at the end of proper evaluation.

References

Arntz A: Treatment of borderline personality disorder: a challenge for cognitive-behavioural therapy. Behav Res Ther 32:419–430, 1994

Arntz A: Do personality disorders exist? on the validity of the concept and its cognitive-behavioral formulation and treatment. Behav Res Ther 37:S97–S134, 1999

Arntz A, Dietzel R, Dreessen L: Assumptions in borderline personality disorder: specificity, stability and relationship with etiological factors. Behav Res Ther 37:545–557, 1999

Beck AT: Depression: Clinical, Experimental, & Theoretical Aspects. New York, Hoeber, 1967

Beck AT, Emery G, Greenberg RL: Anxiety Disorders and Phobias: A Cognitive Perspective. New York, Basic Books, 1985

Beck AT, Freeman A, et al: Cognitive Therapy of Personality Disorders. New York, Guilford, 1990

Benjamin LS: Special feature. Personality disorders: models for treatment and strategies for treatment development. J Personal Disord 11:307–324, 1997

Black DW, Wesner RB, Gabel J, et al: Predictors of short-term treatment response in 66 patients with panic disorder. J Affect Disord 30:233–241, 1994

Blackburn IM, Davidson K: Cognitive Therapy for Depression and Anxiety; A Practitioner's Guide, 2nd Edition. Oxford, England, Blackwell Science, 1995, pp 196–197

Chambless DL, Tran GQ, Glass CR: Predictors of response to cognitive-behavioral group therapy for social phobia. J Anxiety Disord 11:221–240, 1997

Crawford MJ, Wessely S: Does initial management affect the rate of repetition of deliberate self harm? a cohort study. BMJ 317:985, 1998

Crosbie J: Interrupted time-series analysis with brief single-subject data. J Consult Clin Psychol 61:966–974, 1993

Davidson K: Cognitive Therapy for Personality Disorders: A Clinician's Guide. Oxford, England, Butterworth-Heinemann, 2000

Davidson K, Tyrer P: Cognitive therapy for antisocial and borderline personality disorder: single case study series. Br J Clin Psychol 35:413–429, 1996

de Haan E, van Oppen P, van Balkom AJ, et al: Prediction of outcome and early vs late improvement in OCD patients treated with cognitive behaviour therapy and pharmacotherapy. Acta Psychiatr Scand 96:354–361, 1997

Dreessen L, Hoekstra R, Arntz A: Personality disorders do not influence the results of cognitive and behavior therapy for obsessive compulsive disorder. J Anxiety Disord 11:503–521, 1997

Evans K, Tyrer P, Catalan J, et al: Manual-assisted cognitive-behaviour therapy (MACT): a randomised controlled trial of a brief intervention with bibliotherapy in the treatment of recurrent deliberate self-harm. Psychol Med 29:19–25, 1999

Fyer MR, Frances AJ, Sullivan T, et al: Co-morbidity of borderline personality disorder. Arch Gen Psychiatry 45:348–352, 1988

Griggs SMLB, Tyrer PJ: Personality disorder, social adjustment and treatment outcome in alcoholics. J Stud Alcohol 42:802–805, 1981

Hardy GE, Barkham M, Shapiro DA, et al: Impact of Cluster C personality disorders on outcomes of contrasting brief psychotherapies for depression. J Consult Clin Psychol 63:997–1004, 1995

Hersen M, Barlow DH: Single Case Experimental Designs: Strategies for Studying Behavior. New York, Pergamon, 1976

Hiller W, Zaudig M, Mombour W, et al: Munich Diagnostic Checklist for DSM-III-R Axis II. Munich, Germany, Institute of Psychiatry, University of Munich, 1991

Kingdon D, Turkington D, John C: Cognitive behaviour therapy of schizophrenia. Br J Psychiatry 164:581–587, 1994

Kingdon D, Tyrer P, Seivewright N, et al: The Nottingham Study of Neurotic Disorder: influence of cognitive therapists on outcome. Br J Psychiatry 169:93–97, 1996

Linehan MM: Cognitive Therapy for Borderline Personality Disorder. New York, Guilford, 1992

Links PS, Heslegrave R, van Reekum R: Prospective follow-up study of borderline personality disorder: prognosis, prediction of outcome, and axis II comorbidity. Can J Psychiatry 43:265–270, 1998

Longabaugh R, Rubin A, Malloy P, et al: Drinking outcomes of alcohol abusers diagnosed as antisocial personality disorder. Alcohol Clin Exp Res 18:778–785, 1994

Macleod AK, Tata P, Evans K, et al: Recovery of positive future thinking within a high-risk suicide group: results from a pilot randomized controlled trial. Br J Clin Psychol 37:371–379, 1998

Mulhall DJ: Systematic self-assessment by PQRST: Personal Questionnaire Rapid Scaling Technique. Psychol Med 6:591–597, 1976

Nishith P, Mueser KT, Srsic CS, et al: Differential response to cognitive therapy in parolees with primary and secondary substance use disorders. J Nerv Ment Dis 185:763–766, 1997

Patience DA, McGuire RJ, Scott AI, et al: The Edinburgh Primary Care Depression Study: personality disorder and outcome. Br J Psychiatry 167:324–330, 1995

Peck DF: Research with single (or few) patients, in Research Methods in Psychiatry: A Beginner's Guide, 2nd Edition. Edited by Freeman C, Tyrer P. London, England, Gaskell Books, Royal College of Psychiatrists, 1992, pp 82–97

Salkovskis PM, Atha C, Storer D: Cognitive-behavioural problem solving in the treatment of patients who repeatedly attempt suicide: a controlled trial. Br J Psychiatry 157:871–876, 1990

Sanislow CA, McGlashan TH: Treatment outcome of personality disorders. Can J Psychiatry 43:237–250, 1998

Shea MT: Standardised approaches to individual therapy of patients with borderline personality disorder. Hospital and Community Psychiatry 42:1034–1038, 1991

Stone MB: Treatment of borderline patients: a pragmatic approach. Psychiatr Clin North Am 13:265–285, 1990

Tarrier N, Wittkowski A, Kinney C, et al: Durability of the effects of cognitive-behavioural therapy in the treatment of chronic schizophrenia: 12-month follow-up. Br J Psychiatry 174:500–504, 1999

Tyrer P, Seivewright N, Ferguson B, et al: The Nottingham Study of Neurotic Disorder: relationship between personality status and symptoms. Psychol Med 20:423–431, 1990

Tyrer P, Seivewright N, Ferguson B, et al: The Nottingham Study of Neurotic Disorder: effect of personality status on response to drug treatment, cognitive therapy and self-help over two years. Br J Psychiatry 162:219–226, 1993

Tyrer P, Gunderson J, Lyons M, et al: Extent of comorbidity between mental state and personality disorders. J Personal Disord 11:242–259, 1997

Warwick HM: A cognitive-behavioural approach to hypochondriasis and health anxiety. J Psychosom Res 33:705–711, 1989

Warwick HMC, Clark DM, Cobb AM, et al: A controlled trial of cognitive-behavioural treatment of hypochondriasis. Br J Psychiatry 169:189–195, 1996

World Health Organization: International Statistical Classification of Diseases and Related Health Problems, 10th Revision. Geneva, World Health Organization, 1992

Young JE: Cognitive Therapy for Personality Disorders: A Schema-Focused Approach. Sarasota, FL, Professional Resource Exchange, 1990

Young JE: Cognitive Therapy for Personality Disorders: A Schema-Focused Approach, Revised Edition (Practitioners Resource Series). Sarasota, FL, Professional Resource Press, 1994

Zigmond AS, Snaith RP: The Hospital Anxiety and Depression Scale. Acta Psychiatr Scand 57:361–370, 1983

Afterword

Glen O. Gabbard, M.D.
John G. Gunderson, M.D.

What can we conclude from this overview of psychotherapy for personality disorders? First, in an era when psychopharmacology can dominate discussions of therapeutics in the specialty of psychiatry, psychotherapy remains the major modality for this diagnostic group. Second, although managed care companies and insurance companies often claim that they do not cover psychotherapy for personality disorders because no evidence indicates that such treatment works, a growing empirical literature suggests that patients with many personality disorders do indeed benefit from psychotherapy. Moreover, although we have not emphasized it in the chapters of this volume, accumulating evidence also indicates that in some cases psychotherapy is a highly cost-effective treatment for personality disorders (Gabbard et al. 1997; Heard 1994; Stevenson and Meares 1999).

Despite these promising results, research on psychotherapy for personality disorders is still in its early stages. As the review by Perry and Bond (see Chapter 1) illustrates, there is a paucity of randomized controlled trials that rigorously demonstrate the efficacy of specific psychotherapeutic treatments for particular personality disorders. In some of the trials that do exist, it is difficult to determine whether receiving *more* treatment than the control group was the crucial outcome factor or whether it was the *specificity* of the particular psychotherapeutic treatment provided. In addition, we do not know as much as we would like to about the optimal length of treatment. Studying extended psychotherapy of Axis II disorders presents formidable challenges, including suitable controls, intervening life events, the complication of Axis I or medical disorders, and the potential for high dropout rates.

Another conclusion that can be drawn from this overview is that although psychotherapy is central, treatment teams involving multiple treaters often are involved in the overall treatment plan.

In Chapter 3, Gabbard illustrates how pharmacotherapy may be useful as an adjunct to psychotherapy. By addressing underlying temperament, targeting specific personality disorder symptoms, or treating comorbid Axis I conditions, these agents may foster a state of mind in the patient that makes that patient more amenable to psychotherapeutic efforts. In Chapter 2, Gunderson stresses the importance of clearly designating the primary clinician as the person who oversees the treatment plan and is responsible for the safety of patients with borderline personality disorder. Both Gabbard and Gunderson comment on the increasingly common practice of "split treatment," in which different functions are assigned to different treaters. Coordination of these multiple treatments becomes crucial.

In Chapter 4, Stone suggests that considerable caution must be exercised when prescribing treatment for patients with antisocial personality disorder. Particularly useful is the distinction between psychopathy and antisocial personality disorder. As with other personality disorders, the spectrum of antisocial patients varies from the untreatable to some who may be *somewhat* treatable in certain circumstances. Although psychotherapy with antisocial patients is a proposition entailing much uncertainty, the time series analyses of single cases of borderline personality disorder and antisocial personality disorder patients reported in Chapter 5 by Tyrer and Davidson offer hope that some of these patients may be salvageable.

Finally, the treatability of personality disorders with psychotherapy may help psychiatry rethink its traditional view of Axis II conditions. A distinction that has historically been made between Axis I disorders and personality disorders is that the former are ego-*dystonic* conditions that create subjective distress within the patient, whereas the latter are considered ego-*syntonic* conditions and therefore are more likely to create distress in others. However, the fact that so many patients with personality disorders avail themselves of psychotherapy and continue with it long enough to benefit from the treatment suggests that these patients do indeed have significant distress. The recognition of the suffering inherent in personality disorders may ultimately help treaters to take a more empathic perspective to this large group of patients encountered in daily psychiatric practice.

References

Gabbard GO, Lazar SG, Hornberger J, et al: The economic impact of psychotherapy: a review. Am J Psychiatry 154:147–155, 1997

Heard H: Behavior therapies for borderline patients. Paper presented at the 147th annual meeting of the American Psychiatric Association, Philadelphia, PA, May 21–26, 1994

Stevenson J, Meares R: Psychotherapy with borderline patients, II: a preliminary cost benefit study. Aust N Z J Psychiatry 33:473–477, 1999

Index

*Page numbers printed in **boldface** type refer to tables or figures.*